I0447376

iheartmyLaser

Cold Laser Technology & Frequency Healing

Carmen Harris

Space-for-Grace Publishing

"Many things inexplicable a thousand years ago are no longer so, and matters mysterious now may become lawfully intelligible a few years hence."

Paramahansa Yogananda

For My Family
R, N, M, J

About the Author

✳✳✳

Carmen, a Sociology graduate (BA Hons, London University) began her career in community theatre, establishing her own theatre company as a vehicle for her plays. Deciding it was time to get a 'proper' job, she later became a Resources Manager in a psychology-based business consultancy. In this supportive and creative environment she was able to further develop her artistic skills, writing corporate training materials that included audio and video scripts.

During this period, she found the time to author several children's books (Heinemann / Orchard Books). After winning a comedy-writing competition, she went on to become a radio and TV scriptwriter, using the pseudonym Lisselle Kayla. Her past work includes a number of BBC commissions in children's drama, sitcoms and soaps. This track record comprises 2 series of her own original primetime BBC1 sitcom, 'Us Girls,' as well as 10 years as a core writer for the UK's premier TV soap.

She has always had an intense interest in the mind/body field, acquiring an extensive library of books and attending countless workshops. Her life changed dramatically in later years when an experience with a friend's terminally ill daughter led her to realise her innate healing abilities. She now combines creative writing with important work as an intuitive healer and certified practitioner.

She currently lives in London with her partner and two younger children, and near her adult daughter.

The information in this book is not intended to diagnose, prescribe or treat. The details contained herein should in no way be considered as a substitute for the care and advice of a duly licensed healthcare professional

CONTENTS

TESTIMONIAL

The placement of the two lasers at various points on my neck and back at first felt, very simply, like the application of a good, gentle pressure. Not unlike having someone's hand gently resting on your back. Lying face-down, I felt the entire length of my body settling into itself. It was very relaxing, and at the same time fortifying - especially as I became more and more aware of the energy emanating from the lasers. As Carmen periodically changed the settings and positions of the lasers, I felt different areas opening, strengthening, and aligning in new ways. When I turned onto my back, face-up, I didn't feel exposed but instead felt immersed in a space that was at once sheltering and freshening. In addition to the steady energy from the lasers, I became aware of other sources of energy cohering at critical points, especially around my cranium - the work of Carmen's hands. During this time, I felt my body coming into a powerful equilibrium. I also felt a gathering mental clarity. When Carmen asked me questions, I had no trouble producing responses; normally, however, I am prone to over-think; my head gets in the way when a candid response is called for. Not so in this case. To my great surprise, I also experienced a rapid flow of positive memories, from many stages of my life, prompted by the images Carmen asked me to call up (I learned this was evident to her, as well, from my rapid eye movement). Also to my great surprise, my stomach (the site of my medical problems) was responding quite audibly, making noises, sorting and resorting in a profound way. I experienced this gastrointestinal activity as another form of opening, realigning, and grounding. The session ended as gently as it had begun, but I felt strongly altered. In fact, not too long afterwards I fell asleep — had a kind of a deep power-nap for 45 minutes -something I'm usually not able to accomplish when I need it and have the chance. I awoke feeling a great sense of coherence and well-being.

P.S. I need to say again how amazed I am that you mentioned my spleen, first thing. I can't tell you how many years (2+) and tests it took, before my doctors brought that up as a possibility.

Caryn (from California, visiting the UK)

PREFACE

First of all, let me make it clear. I am writing this book from the perspective of a regular, everyday person. I am not a multi-millionaire (so far), I count only five digits on the ends of each of my limbs, I've never been able to fire-walk or breathe flames of fire, my background is of uneventful descent, and I'm currently raising a normal family in a comfortable but typical neighbourhood. However, by virtue of what I do, partly for a living, some of you may consider me as being far from ordinary. You see, I believe in something that many would argue does not exist. I operate within a realm that is apparently invisible and *imperceptible* to the ordinary senses. I work with energy – not the type derived from fossil fuel, but the type that is commonly referred to as '*aura*.' I am a professional writer, but I am also an intuitive healer.

I can already sense a few sceptical twitches among you, dear readers. I may even have spooked those of you with low levels of 'woo-woo' tolerance. Well, if this is all sounding a little too challenging for your belief system let me assure you: like you, I too am a healthy sceptic. Though deeply spiritual, I am not religious in any sense (but I do have great respect for the original aim of all World Religions to unite humanity with a Higher Source), so I do not, and never have, subscribed to 'blind faith.' Any new idea or product that comes my way, I must first connect with it – either logically in the head, or viscerally in the gut. After that, I demand actual proof that the thing does what it promises on the tin. If that idea or thing fails to deliver or live up to my expectations of it, I do not hang around for too long. In short, I am a little impatient. I am also not the kind of person who takes to wafting around in white, incense-smelling robes, waving my arms in the air for creative effect. That would be just plain stupid (not to mention embarrassing); not to mention clearly fraudulent (if I am accepting money for healing as opposed to empty-arm-waving services). And in case you're still not buying any of this 'healer/healing' nonsense, neither am I delusional. When last I checked my mental status, I was firmly on the right side of sane – whatever sanity means these days.

Having said all of this, when I had my first experience of a cold laser, I was not in charge of my critical faculties, nor in any position to exercise my usual uber-scepticism. I was in extreme pain and reduced to dumbly submitting myself to the low level light treatment (LLLT) on offer. The *proof* of the laser's efficacy became clear when the back pain that had held me in a vice for weeks, within minutes, magically loosened its hold, and I could breathe again. Nothing else had come close to giving me the kind of relief that I experienced beneath those Red, Infrared and Violet diodes. It was only weeks later, gratefully relieved of my sole preoccupation with pain, that I started looking into the mechanics of this wonderful technology. My findings both startled and excited me.

I began to understand the direct connection between the energy that emanates from the beams of these cold lasers and the energy flowing from the chakras in the palm of my hands when healing. This was my starting point to writing this book. I saw a fascinating opportunity to not only inform cold laser users how to obtain the greatest benefits from their device, but also to educate those who care to listen, about the field from which the laser's energy is drawn. Here, I might add, that I may give the impression of being knowledgeable of scientific matters, but allow me to make another thing clear: I am not a physicist. I am not even scientifically literate. As I said earlier, I am a fairly standard human specimen. But for the fact that, along the way, I woke up and came to the realisation of something quite profound: *actually, we are extraordinary human beings.* There is so much more to us than meets the eye – or any of our five senses. We are Quantum beings connected to a Quantum Universe. Now, this may sound like empty spiritual warblings to some of you, but my aim within these pages is to convince you otherwise. You see, after experiencing the cold laser, in a very practical and realistic sense, I was even more drawn towards the Quantum field – that invisible force that gives life and vitality to every single molecule, atom, and subatomic particle in every single living thing in the entire Universe. I saw before me an amazing opportunity:

- To help bring the vocation of healing out of its dark, mysterious and cobwebbed 'woo-woo' closet;

- To demonstrate the scientific/spiritual marriage in the awesome magic that these cold lasers can achieve;

- To convince you that each one of us has the power of attaining health and healing when we acknowledge and embrace the energy field that surrounds us all.

I'd like to think that this book, in part, is your own wake-up call: to recognise your vast untapped potential, the key to which lies outside the illusion of this, our 'material' world.

So, to those of you whom I have not yet sent screaming for the safety of the distant hills, let me begin...

INTRODUCTION

WHY I WROTE THIS HANDBOOK

SIMPLY PUT

I have written this Handbook from the perspective of both a cold laser user and an intuitive healer. I have treated numerous friends and clients presenting varying conditions – either solely using a cold laser, without using the laser, or combining use of the laser.

As a healer, I DO NOT claim to have medical expertise, nor give any such advice. My work is always complementary to, and never in conflict with, the professional and allopathic guidance already given to my clients.

This Handbook is based entirely on my passion for the cold laser and my personal viewpoint and experience of using it. Any suggestions in this Handbook should be taken at your own discretion.

FDA Cleared for aching joints, muscle pains, to increase blood circulation, and relax muscles.

***

Indicated for temporary relief of minor muscle, joint and arthritic pain, muscle spasm and stiffness, promoting relaxation of muscle tissue, and to temporarily increase local blood circulation.

Anyone who uses a cold laser and who reads disclaimers such as those above must surely be aware that these descriptions fall far short of their laser's true capabilities. Personal anecdotes of healing and rejuvenation proliferate the internet. Surely that many ordinary people (myself included) would not waste their precious time and energy submitting unfounded or misleading testimonials, just for the sake of it? No, of course not.

It is obvious that the advertised potential of this wonderful technology has been limited to what it has *scientifically* been proven to achieve. We are all familiar, however, with the rigours of empirical scientific validation. Years, sometimes decades, of rounds of exhaustive investigation, verification and peer review means that the full appreciation of a fresh method or an innovative new product such as the cold laser can often lag far behind personal evidence and experience. Further in this book I'll be giving historical examples of how certain 'solid' scientific 'facts' later gave way to more advanced knowledge about our Universe. But only after the proponents of these new ideas were first ridiculed and rejected.

The Chinese were applying the art of acupuncture for thousands of years before we in the West finally got around to taking notice. Science is now cautiously satisfied of the efficacy of fine needles inserted into certain points in the body to alleviate a range of medical conditions. As an intuitive healer, I am able to feel a person's aura and detect corresponding issues in the body. I once held my hand a foot away from the chest of an acquaintance (who would later become a client). I felt a piercing discomfort in my palm, which he confirmed he could feel as intense heat in the centre of his chest. The sensation coming from his *heart chakra* was so strong I was in no doubt that he had a real issue to do with his heart. His reply came as no surprise. He said he'd been hospitalised four years prior after having had a heart attack. I'd had no previous knowledge of this. Simply from the 'feel' of his aura, I was picking up that his heart was still in poor condition. A scientist would dispute this event could be possible, or that such a thing as a detectable aura exists.

One day the same will be true of the cold laser. The scientists who now claim that its functions are limited to the temporary relief of minor ailments will come round to telling us what we already know. Those of us who use cold lasers recognise without hesitation that its benefits go far beyond its statutorily limited claims. And for anyone suffering now, it may be felt that one really doesn't have the luxury of waiting for science to catch up. Profound and permanent transformation can be achieved by the cold laser. We already know this. Below is my very first wave of healing experiences using my new cold laser:

- o I run a monthly Meetup group to teach healing techniques and encourage others to take responsibility for their own healing. Several times I have invited Arram, a friend, to demonstrate the cold laser to the group. On this occasion there were two women present, both called Celia, and both suffering from **severe arthritis** that caused them pain 24/7. At the outset they individually rated their pain an unreserved 10 out of 10. I watched them moving my laser over various parts of their body. Twenty minutes later, the first Celia said her pain had gone down to 5; whilst the second Celia's pain had reduced to 4. What was interesting was that the first Celia, when asked initially how she was doing, replied impatiently that the pain in her left foot had gone completely but there was still some pain in one knee. I suggested that she might want to give thanks to the foot that was now pain-free! I found it interesting because it demonstrates our innate memory of the body's naturally healthy blueprint. Once the body is back in balance, we often quickly forget what it was like when it was out of balance. As for Celia 2, she was bending, stooping and traipsing up and down the stairs in a manner that was completely different to her cautious, crippled posture when she first walked through the door. Her relaxed, smiling face said it all.

o My partner used to complain each time he arrived home from work about the balls of his **feet** really hurting him. Each time he complained I would sit him down on the sofa and instruct him to give himself 10 minutes with the laser on the area. He'd done this about six different times. Then it occurred to me that lately I hadn't heard him complaining. I asked how his feet were. He casually said they were OK. This result was after MONTHS of complaining. At the time of writing, he is still trouble-free.

o We were having dinner with friends when their son (age 15) doubled up in agony with **growing pains** in his thigh. I introduced my laser, and told him to hold it against his leg. Within 8 minutes he said that his leg felt much better. When he walked away from the table, he was pain-free. His mother said that usually his growing pains would hang around for ages till he took pain-killers. I have also used the laser for my own son's growing pains with great success. (Both boys are league footballers).

o My sister came round with her young grandson who'd suffered the **shock** of being run over by a car. Luckily, he escaped with only cuts and bruises. My sister said she could also do with a session. I started with her grandson first and put him on the massage couch and did tapping (EFT) and healing whilst putting the laser on various settings on various parts of his body. He went into a deep and healing two hour sleep during which I was reluctant to move him from the couch. Without the use of the couch I was reluctant to do healing work on my sister (she told me she had a bit of a tummy ache) as I would risk straining my back by bending over too low. Instead, I put the laser on her where she lay, and asked that she come back another time for a full healing session. She too went into a lovely sleep, right there on the sofa. The next day she texted: *'My **stomach** upset has gone which I had for over 2 weeks. I cannot* *believe that it has gone and keep expecting it to come back.'* I'd had no idea her stomach issue had been so long-standing!

o   My **asthmatic** friend came to visit. I was in my bedroom at the top of the house and by the time she climbed all four flights of stairs, she was wheezy and out of breath. When she sat down and reached for her inhaler. I asked her to try the laser instead. Her breathing noticeably relaxed after a few minutes and a few hours later she still had not needed her inhaler. The next day I asked her how she got on and she said that before going to bed, she'd automatically used her puffer as she'd suffered attacks in the past and (quite rightly), wasn't about to risk another one, but it certainly wasn't because she felt breathless or the need for her puffer.

o   I have noticed an amazing by-product of using the laser. My **fingernails** used to be so weak and flaky, I'd regularly have them strengthened with acrylic at the local nail bar. I was aware, however, that long-term this would only weaken them further. After a few months, coinciding with buying and using my laser, I decided to cut my nails short and wear them au naturel. Within weeks, I noticed that they were not as 'spring-boardy' as they used to be. I now wear my own, natural nails at quite a length and they are rock hard - as hard as when I used to coat them with acrylic! The only thing I can put this down to is use of the laser. I now no longer have to pay £30 every three weeks to have them strengthened, and they look beautiful!

o   I'd finished my session with a client when he mentioned that a week prior he'd queued for four hours in the cold to purchase some tickets to a very popular art exhibition. Since then both **knees** had been hurting, but he reckoned this might also have something to do with advancing age, and there wouldn't be much he could do about that. I suggested that he use the laser whilst we were debriefing about the session. Twenty minutes later he said that his knees felt much better. By the time he got his coat and bags and was at the door, he said in amazement that the pain had completely gone from both knees!

o My neighbour was exhausted from a hard week at work. I gave her a quick demonstration session on the laser. She said it made her feel relaxed but desperate to go home to sleep. A few days later I bumped into her. She told me excitedly that when she woke up the next day she was surprised to discover that she was without pain in her **knees**! She reminded me that she'd had an operation on both knees over two years previously and that since then she'd suffered from constant pain. Two weeks later I saw her again and she told me that she was still pain-free. I was just as surprised as she was, as I hadn't used the laser anywhere near her knees!

o *Animals benefit, too!*

My friend's **dog**, Diesel, was poorly. He had myster-iously hurt his **paw** and had been unwell for some days. I had my laser in my bag and Diesel took to it right away. He relaxed contentedly on my lap as I used the laser on his entire body and paw. Later, we went for a walk and my friend commented that Diesel was pulling hard on the lead and seemed to have more energy. On that walk, her son, Jack, caught his finger in an iron gate. He was distressed and crying, and a dark **bruise** appeared. Almost as soon as I put the laser on him, he calmed down, fascinated by the light that the laser was emitting. I used the laser for less than 5 minutes but, half an hour later, after putting ice on Jack's finger, the bruise was barely detectable. My friend wrote: "*Diesel took to his bed clearly absolutely exhausted after your visit. So I was all set to take him to the vet this morning, but his paw seems completely better today, and he is like his old self... he hasn't whimpered or flinched about the paw once. Jack's finger looks like the bruise happened about two weeks ago by the way, not yesterday! Absolutely amazing.*"

> ### SIMPLY PUT
>
> I heart my Laser SO much I decided to write this Handbook to ensure as many people as possible understand how to use their own laser and experience its miraculous benefits.

I should make it clear that I am not being paid to promote any cold laser of any kind. Neither have I ever been approached directly or by any third party associated with any laser company concerning the publication of this Handbook. I am a free agent and laser owner, and as such, I am at liberty to make claims based on my enthusiasm for this technology and my discoveries whilst using it. My main objectives in writing this Handbook* are for three simple reasons. To:

- o Declare that these lasers actually *work*!
- o Demonstrate how the true power of cold lasers go way beyond what is (or even can be) described
- o Make these facts known to as many people as possible.

*I am assuming that the reader is already familiar with the basic functions of their laser such as switching on and off, navigating around the various programmes, and recharging the unit.

I am also assuming that the reader has read their particular cold laser Warnings, Precautions and Contra-indications concerning use.

PART I

CHAPTER 1
HOW TO USE THIS HANDBOOK

SIMPLY PUT

What setting should I choose?
For how long should I apply the setting?
Where on my body should I place the laser?
How many times should I use my laser?

Answer: There is no single answer!

- Some of the instructions in this Handbook are best suited to programmable cold lasers that give the user a wider scope for flexibility and experimentation.

- Some manufacturers give specific directions for their product, but as long as you follow normal sensible precautions (eg. don't aim the laser light at your eyes; first seek medical guidance if you are pregnant or wearing a pace-maker, etc.) there's no harm at all in experimenting. Cold laser energy has been proven to be perfectly safe but, where our health is concerned, it is simply common sense to always err on the side of caution.

- This Handbook is an attempt to <u>clarify</u> and <u>broaden</u> your options, not limit them. You may find that some ideas work for you, and others don't. That's OK. It doesn't mean you've got it wrong, it just means that there's another solution for you. Be creative. Experiment. Go with what FEELS right, and by the RESULTS you achieve. Each one of us is unique and, no matter whether we are suffering from the same medically labelled condition – arthritis; cancer; hyper-tension – our reactions to the condition and our healing from the condition is unlikely to follow an identical path.

- I'm sharing my experience and know-how, but your own intuition is equally valid. Just as there are many different approaches to healing, there are many different combinations and methods of using your laser to give relief and achieve a state of mental and physical balance. The truth is, Laser Light Therapy is not an exact science. We are learning and sharing our experiences all the time: amongst ourselves and with the very people who manufacture these devices.

- Give your healing the *time* it deserves. Some chronic conditions have been created over a long period, sometimes decades. You will need to be patient. I expected my back complaint to be better in a matter of days. Actually, it took several weeks before the deep pain dissolved. And several more weeks for me to feel whole and like my old self again. Even *better* than my old self. But each day that I used my laser, I noticed an incremental improvement. That was encouraging. That became my focus.

- Your mental attitude is so important. Intention is everything. Shift your perspective from 'cup half-empty' to 'cup half-full.' Train your mind to look for signs of progress (eg. less phlegm than the day before; gradual relaxation of stiff muscles; subtle return of energy, more good days than bad days, etc.), rather than focusing (like Celia 1) on signs of non-progress - 'The pain is still there!' The mind plays a major role in assisting our body to recover (that's why placebos work so well!). The person who is persistently disgruntled and expecting the worst will have a harder time recovering than the person who is open to the idea that healing is on its way, or that health is the body's natural state.

CHAPTER 2
LASER FACTS

1916:   Though **Albert Einstein** did not invent the laser, his work laid the foundations when he conceived the theory of *Light Amplification through Stimulated Emission* of *Radiation* (**LASER**).

1967:   **Prof. Andre Mester** (Budapest, Hungary) has become known as the 'grandfather of laser therapy.' He began using low power lasers to treat non-healing wounds and ulcers in diabetic patients. His 70% success rate led to the development of the science of what he called *Laser Bio-stimulation*.

- Whereas an ordinary lightbulb's energy is diffuse, a laser emits an intense beam of **coherent** light. Its parallel beam is able to concentrate light energy to small diameters.

- Anything over 500mW has thermal (ie heat-generating) potential. 'Hot' lasers that cut, burn and cauterise, deliver power from 1mW to 500mW. The energy output of cold lasers, however, is well **below one Watt of energy**.

- The 'Cold laser' is commonly referred to by **other terms** - Soft Laser, Low Power Laser, Bio-stimulation Laser, Therapeutic Laser, Low Level Laser, (LLLT stands for Low Level Light Therapy), etc.

SIMPLY PUT

Since 1967 there have been thousands of clinical studies published worldwide. Many of these studies are double-blinded, placebo-controlled and have demonstrated cold laser therapy to be a proven method for pain relief.

David Rindge (HealingLightsSeminars.com) has compiled an amazing Laser Research Library.
It contains an impressive and continually updated number of peer-reviewed scientific studies from around the world on the benefits of Cold Laser Therapy.

- On the market there are **many types and adaptations** of cold lasers and how they are used – from portable, hand-held devices, to large units for the whole body; from laser caps and laser combs to regenerate hair, to pen lasers and probes

used in acupuncture treatment; from lasers that cost several
hundred pounds/dollars, to those that would set you back tens
of thousands; from fixed protocol lasers, to user-
programmable lasers; from LED lasers to what are known as
*'true' lasers, and lasers that combine the technology of both.

LASERS vs. LEDs

*A true laser focuses all of its energy in one direction
in a very concentrated line, delivering as much as 90%
of power to the treatment area.

LED devices (which can use red and infrared light)
are usually cheaper than true lasers, have beneficial
effects, and cover a wider area than a single laser
beam. They are, however, limited to the treatment of
tissue at superficial levels.

Laser researchers agree that laser light therapy is far
superior to LED therapy.

LED = Light Emitting Diodes

*Diodes = component that allows an electric current to
travel in a single direction*

- A wide range of **professionals** use cold lasers (in the past,
  almost exclusively), including chiropractors, physical
  therapists, medical doctors, naturopathic doctors, osteopaths,

acupuncturists, veterinarians, dentists, podiatrists, sports therapists, and massage therapists.

Treatment claims of Cold Lasers include:

Increased/accelerated:

- Blood circulation
- Body's ability to handle stress
- Cell reproduction and growth
- Cellular energy
- Collagen and elastin
- Endorphins (body's natural pain killers)
- Healing enzymes
- Immune response
- Lymphatic drainage
- Nerve function /nerve cell reconnection
- Oxygen and food particle loads to cells
- Speed of bone repair
- Wound healing

Decreased / elimination of:

- Fibrous (scar) tissue formation
- Joint stiffness
- Muscle spasms
- Swelling
- Viruses, fungi, bacteria, parasites

Advertised benefits include:

- o Relieves acute and chronic pain
- o Increases the speed, quality and tensile strength of tissue repair
- o Increases blood supply
- o Stimulates immune system
- o Stimulates nerve function
- o Develops collagen and muscle tissue
- o Helps generate new and healthy cells and tissue

Advertised conditions treated include:

- o Acute and chronic pain
- o Arthritis
- o Back pain
- o Bursitis
- o Carpal Tunnel Syndrome
- o Fibromyalgia
- o Ligament sprains
- o Muscle strain
- o Soft tissue injuries
- o Tendonitis
- o Tennis elbow

Cold Laser Variability:

- Basic **features** vs. multi-functional?
- Set **protocols** vs user-programmable?
- Low, middle, or high **power** (mW)?
- Continuous **wave** vs. Pulsed or Superpulsed? The latter both deliver more power and deeper penetration, but this is not necessarily a 'better' option. It all depends on your issue. A continuous wave relaxes/sedates the cell, reduces inflammation and kills pain. Pulsed light stimulates the cell to produce protein and speed up healing.
- **Power**? – Lower power (eg. 5mW per diode) is good for unwinding stress; Higher power is good for driving photons deeper and faster into the body and for acupuncture points.
- Small and portable or larger in **size**?
- **Probe**/pen-laser vs. probe attachment(s) to a main unit?
- Quantity of **diodes** – single/multiple? (the more diodes the larger the treatment area)
- **Price**?

Lasers are designed to help you deal with states and conditions relating to all the cells, organs, glands and systems of the body. Taking your time to learn your laser's functions and how it can personally benefit *you* is all part of your voyage of discovery. I hope the following explanation of laser terminology and use will assist in increasing your understanding and enjoyment of your laser.

CHAPTER 3

THE KILLER LURKING AMONG US

The Number One killer in today's society is no longer the ten-ton dinosaur prowling the pre-historic cave (OK, I hear you – outside of the movies, man and dinosaur never actually co-existed. But in terms of scary beasts, the dinosaur neatly illustrates my point so I'll continue with my analogy). No. According to the acclaimed cellular biologist, Bruce Lipton, the scourge of our times is that familiar state of being: Stress.

Stress, the body's way of responding to pressure, demand or change, is the single common factor behind many diseases and chronic conditions. Over 90% of all health challenges are stress-related. It's true that a little stress never did anyone any harm. In fact, motivational stress ('eu-stress') is healthy, necessary and beneficial. It can make the difference between passing an exam and failing; it can help us get up the courage to talk in front of an audience; it can assist us in meeting a deadline or competing to win a race; or it can enable us to move quickly and successfully out of a dangerous situation. This kind of single-event-related stress isn't the kind that we need to worry about.

We live in a toxic environment. From the brain-zapping mobile technology we press to our ear 24/7, to the fume-filled, train-delayed, traffic-choked, clock-watching journey we make to work each day; to the slights and humiliations and challenges we face in our everyday lives - we are continually being bombarded by stress factors that compromise our total wellbeing.

TYPES OF STRESS	
Outer Physical	Travel; Long work hours; Intense exertion; Sleep deprivation; Pesticides; Radiation; Household chemicals; Industrial chemicals; Extreme temperatures; Noise pollution; etc.
Inner Physical	Food Allergies; Vitamin deficiency; Mineral deficiency; Mercury poisoning; Hunger; Drug dependency; Alcohol abuse; etc.
Traumatic	Injuries; Accidents; Surgery; Illness; Infections; etc
Mental/Emotional	Anger; Guilt; Loneliness; Blame; Shame; Sadness; Fear; Grief; Perfectionism; Worry; Anxiety; etc.
Psycho-spiritual	Relationships issues; Financial pressures; Career worries; Spiritual alignment; General state of happiness; Life goal challenges; etc.

Bruce Lipton's argument likens our cellular make-up to an on/off (binary) switch. When the body is in balance and switched ON, it is functioning normally, and doing what it was primarily designed to do – heal, repair, grow and maintain itself. A state of *homeostasis*. When the body is under stress, however, it becomes imbalanced as the cells' normal functions switch OFF and divert to a fight/flight/ freeze mode of survival. In this state, homeostasis resources are directed away from 'non-vital' functions (digesting, logical thinking, immunity against germs, etc.) as the body is flooded with 'fast response' chemicals - cortisol, adrenaline, and other stress hormones.

This chemical reaction served us well in the days when we were being challenged by Tyranosaurus Rex: a huge spurt of adrenaline-fuelled energy could deliver us from the clutches of danger and the abysmal fate of becoming dino-feed. In today's society, however, the stress response has become a toxic everyday over-reaction to less than life-threatening situations. How many times in a day do you find your heart racing, your brain 'going numb,' your stomach churning, your muscles stiffening? And for what kinds of reason? You glance at your watch and notice that you're half an hour late for work; you hear depressing news being broadcast on the radio or TV; you're at the receiving end of someone's cutting remark; you discover that you've put on a few extra pounds in weight and can no longer fit into your skinny jeans.

This kind of low-grade, 'high-alert' stress, is affecting all of us, minute-by-minute, every day. As time goes by, our exhausted cells, scrambling from one 'emergency' situation to another, start failing to communicate effectively with one another. Headaches, joint pains, hair loss, bad breath, muscle tension, indigestion, frequent colds, depression, irritability, and insomnia are just some of the signs that the body is no longer at ease with itself. Before long, the more serious stuff starts showing up. From 'dis-ease,' we enter the realm of 'disease.' Stress in everyday life is no joke. It is literally a matter of life and death.

This is where your cold laser sails into the picture, and to the rescue. Working at the cellular level, your laser's technology helps to unwind the damaging effects of stress, returning the body to its normal blueprint of homeostasis. How? By communicating with the body via the language of the cells: the language of Light. *Light* = *Energy*.

WHAT IS ENERGY?

Stop for a moment. Rub your hands briskly together for half a minute or so. Now, hold them a hands' span apart, palms-facing. Close your eyes. Engage your senses. Notice what you notice. Do you sense a little pressure between your palms? Some tingling, maybe? Electricity, perhaps? Resistance? Heat? Tension? Heaviness? Play with the space between your palms by slowly and gently pulling your hands apart and drawing them closer together, without touching. The sensations you are feeling is *subtle energy*. Depending on your sensitivity, you will feel this energy to a greater or lesser extent.

This electro-magnetism, or **aura**, surrounds and inter-penetrates everything in the Universe - animate and inanimate, matter and anti-matter - including ourselves. As I move my hands and scan my clients' 'energy fields' this aura is exactly what I am detecting. There's a very important reason for this scanning. I'm certainly not arm-waving simply to 'look the part' of a healer. When we are emotionally, physically or spiritually out of sorts, the imbalance first shows up, not in the physical body, but in the energetic frequency of the person, their aura. This aura is **vibrational energy.**

__Scientific Fact__: We are electro-magnetic beings. Electro-magnetism permeates and surrounds us. This electro-magnetism is measurable and can provide important indicators about the state of our health.

Do I again sense a little nervousness among some of you, my readers? Are those your antennae's standing on end, wary of being lured into the dubious world of this wacky healer? Well, consider this for a second. If you've ever been to hospital for some kind of diagnosis, chances are you will have undergone at least one of these medical (ie scientific) procedures:

MRI	(electro-magnetic scanner, safer and more effective than x-ray)
EEG/MEG	(records the brain's electrical activity)
ECG/EKG	(measures the heart's electrical activity)
UltraSound	(high frequency sound waves to view internal organs/foetus; pulverise kidney stones, etc.)

Each of these machines measures the electro-magnetic frequency emanating from our cells.

Remember the energy 'field' between the palm of your hands? Think of the healer scanning the aura of his or her client. This electro-magnetism is detectable, and its frequencies can be manipulated to bring about beneficial cellular change. This is what laser technology is designed to do. This is what healers have been doing since time began. Science and spirituality are converging. Your laser is at the interface between two seemingly irreconcilable worlds.

LIGHT AND COLOUR

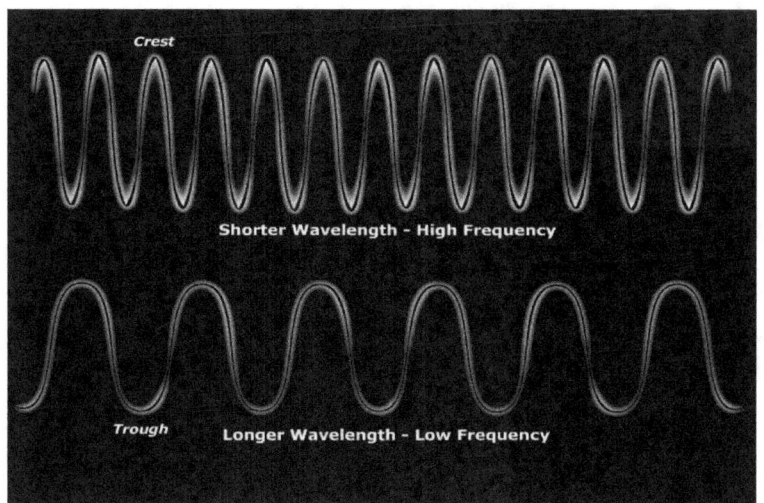

Steve Thorne

- Light (photons) travels by oscillating in a *wavelike* motion.

- The number of oscillations (up-and-down, wave-like, movements) per second, is referred to as *frequency*.

- The measurement from the peak (or crest) of one wave to another is called a *wavelength*.

- Shorter wavelengths oscillate faster (takes less time for the wave pattern to repeat itself)

- Longer wavelengths oscillate more slowly (crests are farther apart)

SIMPLY PUT

Light occurs in wavelengths and those wavelengths are measured in nanometers (nm).

1nm= one billionth of a meter.

All levels of light can have biological effect on the cells, whether detrimental or therapeutic. Think of the sun's rays stimulating Vitamin D (good), or causing skin cancer (bad). Think of the caution advised regarding exposure to the UV lights of tanning machines. Think of blue light therapy used to successfully treat jaundice in newborns.

Light is one type of electro-magnetic wave, and contains all the colours in the electro-magnetic spectrum. Colour is frequency within the *visible* portion of the spectrum. Whilst at either ends of this electro-magnetic spectrum we find the *invisible* realms of infrared and ultraviolet. Each wave vibrates at a certain frequency, and each colour is composed of a band of frequencies.

VISIBLE spectrum of Light (Colour)	380 – 760nm
Violet/Blue light (visible)	380 – 420nm
Red light (visible)	630 – 670nm
Infrared light (invisible)	760nm (& above)

NB: Wavelength (nm) determines how deep the photons
(waves/particles of light) go, and what tissues absorb them

*Research has shown that the cells of our body communicate with each other through coherent (steady, uniform) light. Our cells respond to different pulses of frequency by emitting light of a similar frequency (resonance), and returning dysfunctional tissue to a normal level.

*Physicist and biophoton researcher, Prof. Fritz-Albert Popp

<u>SIMPLY PUT</u>

Colour (visible/invisible) = **Light** = ENERGY

<u>Wavelengths</u>   <u>Hertz</u> (Hz)

(measured in nm)   (unit of vibrational frequency)

Energy output (power) measured in mW

Shorter wavelength = HIGHER energy output
LONGER wavelength = **lower** energy output

<u>Visible Wavelengths:</u>
VIOLET - *shortest* wavelength / **RED** – *longest* wavelength

...Violet...Blue...Green....Yellow....Orange....Red.......**Infrared........Ultraviolet....**
..............................*visible*.............................*/...............invisible.................*

Scientific Fact: *30% of sunlight is in the 'healing' red and near-infrared range (630nm to 900nm). These vibrating wavelengths pass through the blood and water in tissue.*

One of the best ways to deliver light into the bloodstream is through the belly button – the aorta artery being behind the navel. After 20 minutes, all the white, red, B and T cell activity will be increased, boosting the immune system.

Your laser's **630-660nm** range (ie visible Red light) is the most advantageous for treating problems close to the surface of the skin (penetrating ¼ - ½ inch) – wounds, cuts, scars; as well as for trigger and acupuncture points.

__Scientific Fact__: The average wavelength of cell tissue in the human body ranges between 600nm and 720 nm; 660nm is the mid-point. 660 nm works better than any other single frequency because it resonates closest to the frequency of cell tissue. It also absorbs better in haemoglobin.

The **760-905nm** range (invisible Infrared) laser delivers energy faster and the beam penetrates deeper (1-3 inches), making it more effective for treating organs and providing relief for ailments of bones, joints and deep muscle tissue.

The biological effects of both ranges are similar:

- oxygenation of the cell
- detoxification of the cell
- absorption of photons by the mitochondria (converted into ATP*)
- DNA replication
- regeneration of damaged nerve tissue.
- cellular metabolism
- activation of endorphins and beneficial enzymes
- deactivation of inflammation-causing enzymes

---

*ATP and MITOCHONDRIA

Your cola laser donates energy (photons) to the cells by stimulating the mitochondria to produce ATP.

Mitochondria - 'little' organ (organelle) that manufactures ATP.

ATP - *'energy currency'* of the cell. Detoxifies cells, tissues and organs of waste products; and repairs, regenerates and rebuilds.

Digested food is converted to ATP in order to extract energy from it. (Plants photosynthesise ATP from sunlight.)

405nm (Violet) frequency:

The violet spectrum is a feature in more advanced cold lasers. Violet has far reaching health and regenerative benefits. It is particularly effective at: a) promoting key enzymes within the cell such as the telomerase enzyme (imagine a glue-like substance, holding our chromosomes together), and b) activating the DNA sequencing for anti-aging and rejuvenation.

1930's - Telomeres first discovered. The ends of human chromosomes found to have structures that prevent different chromosomes from attaching to each other.

1973 - Alexey Olovnikov observed that the ends of human chromosomes shorten with each replication, eventually resulting in DNA replication and cell division permanently ceasing

2009 - Elizabeth Blackburn, Carol Greider and Jack Szostak jointly awarded the Noble Prize in Physiology or Medicine "for the discovery of how chromosomes are protected by telomeres and the enzyme telomerase."

"The connection between cellular aging and telomere length is rooted in solid research. Telomeres become shorter every time a cell divides, and when they are lost cells can no longer reproduce. The enzyme telomerase can lengthen telomeres, possibly slowing or reversing degenerative diseases. In one study, mice genetically engineered to lack functional telomerase showed brain degeneration and shrunken testes, but those effects were reversed when the enzyme was reactivated."

Nature (International Weekly Journal of Science)

"The violet laser helps the body fight off infection at a deeper level and has been shown to help even difficult skin infections. It stimulates the sympathetic nervous system and seems to bring up deeper levels of problems, even stimulating emotional responses to healing. This laser is very useful for patients with chronic long-standing conditions as it seems to find and heal issues on a deeper level."

(Erconia - Cold Laser).

CHAPTER 4

AURA, ZERO-POINT AND SPIRITUALITY

DEVELOPMENT OF THERAPEUTIC USE OF ARTIFICIAL LIGHT

1660's: **Isaac Newton** separated white light (ie sunlight) with a prism and discovered the visible spectrum of colour.

1800:   **William Herschel** studied the temperature of different colours by moving a thermometer through light split by a prism. He noticed that the hottest temperature was beyond the colour red – this could only mean that there was 'light' invisible to the eye. He had discovered infrared.

1801:   **Johann Ritter** working on the other end of the spectrum, discovered that there were light rays beyond visible violet. These 'chemical rays' were renamed ultraviolet radiation.

1890's: **Dr Niels Finsen** observed that tubercular skin lesions were rare in the summer months but much more common during the long dark winter months. Awarded the Nobel prize in 1903, he pioneered light therapy, later using red light to prevent smallpox scars and to treat TB.

The term '**zero point energy**' was first coined in 1913 by *Albert Einstein* and *Otto Stern*. Zero-point describes that all-pervasive, infinite, electro-magnetic field (sometimes referred to as *Stillpoint)* that surrounds and permeates everything: the invisible quantum vibrations of the Universe. Examples of *zero-point* energy are ergon particles, biophoton particles, soliton waves and scalar waves (more of scalar and soliton waves later).

'EMPTY' SPACE

- It used to be thought that after eliminating all matter and all gases, space contained **empty volume** – ie 'empty' space was indeed empty.

- In the late 19th century, it was discovered that 'empty' space actually contained **thermal** (heat) **radiation**.

- It was then theorised that 'empty space' could be achieved by cooling down the vacuum to **zero temperature.**

- Since then, scientists have come to realise that even at absolute zero temperature, the vacuum contains **(non-thermal) radiation.**

- **Your laser** delivers non-thermal radiation.

At our basic physiological level, we are a matrix of vibrating molecules. Everything you can grasp with your five sense organs is composed of these molecules – the building blocks of existence. When matter goes beyond the perception of the five senses but remains physical in nature we are in the area of atoms and sub-atomic particles. Beyond this area - the realm of waves, frequencies and absolute nothingness - our intellect and physical senses cannot help us to discern our own existence.

Traditional approaches to health and healing attempt to address and manipulate issues at our molecular level (ie through the use of prescription drugs). But at our deepest, quantum level, our molecules are also inter-connected with *zero-point* waves or frequencies. In other words, we are permeated and enveloped by a field of vibrating energy (**aura**). These vibrations/frequencies/waves are part of who and what we are, and have an essential impact on our cells. Energy healers like myself, stress our interconnectedness with the Universe or the 'field.' We are all from the *One Source*, whether Adam's rib or the Big Bang. Our aim is always to affect changes at this *quantum* vibratory level.

WE ARE SPIRITUAL BEINGS OF LIGHT

- Science has discovered that photons are both *particles* and *waves*.
- Unaffected by time or distance, photons exist everywhere and all the time ('non-local').
- Photons are an intelligent field linked to our unconscious.

We too are composed of both particles and waves:

Molecules	O
Atoms	o
Subatomic Particles	•

Waves	~

This quantum level is not immediately apparent to us. How could it be, when we experience less than 1% of the Universe we occupy? Our ears, eyes, nose, sense of taste and touch detect only a restricted spectrum of the information that is 'out there.' For example, infrared and ultrasonic sound is outside our visual and audible range and cannot be seen or heard. But we acknowledge and accept that both exist. Some people, however, already have the ability to sense 'extra' signals that most of us cannot detect with our senses. We refer to these people as having 'clair' (ie 'clear') abilities:

clairvoyant	(see)
clairsentient	(sense)
clairaudient	(hear)
clairscentist	(smell)
clairgustant	(taste)
claircognizant	(recognition)

These are those patchouli-scented folk we tend to avoid at parties or ignore in serious conversation: strange creatures who claim to be able to 'see' a person's aura or even into the future. Aside from the obvious charlatans, bogus con-artists and mental asylum escapees, the truth is, these folk have an intellect every bit as functional as yours or mine. The only difference is, they have the additional ability to perceive the subtle frequencies that surround us but are invisible to our 'normal' senses. I understand that most might find this notion way too 'out there' for their particular liking or comfort zone. It does tend to stretch the very bounds of one's imagination. Meanwhile, however, we have no problem accepting the 'magical' images and sounds emanating from our iPads, mobile phones, TV and radio – even though they reach us via frequencies (radio waves) that are inaudible and invisible to the vast majority of us. If we accept that these frequencies do exist, perhaps it wouldn't take much more of a stretch, to accommodate the idea that some of us could be sensitive to them?

Science certainly does not have the monopoly on Truth. Many things in this life remain inexplicable. Nevertheless, we continue to believe that all of existence has to be understood by logic – as though the entire Universe could possibly be accommodated by the limited dimensions of the brain. On the contrary, the brain and our entire physical dimension are accommodated *by* the Universe. In other words, we cannot capture the infinity of the Universe merely by thoughts, or logic alone. Indeed, there are so many occasions when our experience leads us to situations where there is an absence of reassuring certainty – particularly where death or ill health is concerned. Such times often require that we take a leap into our own imagination – allowing intuition, trust, faith, belief and internal guidance to influence us over the presence or otherwise of any 'known facts.'

I hope I've managed to convince you of the plausibility of a boundless, unquantifiable world existing outside of your normal awareness, and that the phenomenon of your aura is a reality. Or, at least you'll trust me enough to stay open to the idea. For, it is this force that determines our health, and must be tapped in order for us to heal. Connected to the *zero-point* energy field, your aura is the essence of who you are. This field of quantum vibrations is responsible for our higher functions of memory, intuition and creativity. One day we will all have the potential to truly become a part of the total reality that envelopes our being. Until such time, your cold laser has the technological ability to transport you to this state, allowing your cells to vibrate at the frequency of *zero-point* energy. At this frequency, we are in the realm of quantum healing. Here, the cells in our bodies are reminded of *Source* - that pain-free, disease-free state they originate from. Returning to this state is the blueprint condition for cellular healing and regeneration.

CHAPTER 5
ADVANCED COLD LASER TECHNOLOGY

NIKOLA TESLA
(1857-1943)

History is littered with examples of the ridicule, contempt and vicious debunking meted out to those who challenged the established 'facts' of the day. Only for the proponents of these new concepts to, over time, then be accepted and their ideas validated. An obvious instance is Galileo's telescope and his 'ludicrous' insistence that the earth circles the sun.

In the margins of our history books you will discover a Serbian called Nikola Tesla. His amazing legacy, starting out as a penniless immigrant to the US, was to invent radio and electrical transmission via a receiver, in place of the use of fossil fuels. Tesla was the true inventor of wireless communication (though Marconi was given the patent). Yet, this outstanding scientist and inventor, operating in the realms of 'sacred science,' died in poverty and isolation, denounced as a crackpot.

In 1899 Tesla demonstrated the existence of a new type of energy: **Scalar energy**. This electromagnetic wave exists in empty space in the 5-dimensional realm and constitutes an ocean of infinite energy. Tesla's vision of harnessing these waves and providing free worldwide energy and communication was dashed by JP Morgan. Morgan, a financier and industrialist, had been backing Tesla but, seeing no profit in providing free energy to mankind, he withdrew his support. After refusing to sell out to such powerful profit-driven interests, Tesla was hounded, persecuted and his work destroyed.

SCALAR ENERGY

Scalar energy is described as zero-frequency (non-Hertzian) energy, always present in the environment, but not existing in the 'material' world. Scalar waves occur in the vacuum of empty space that is all around us as well as existing in and through everything. This vacuum of space, after all, is present even in our bodies, which is mostly empty space between atoms and molecules.

Scalar energy is created when two electromagnetic waves of the same frequency come together from two different vectors or angles and cancel each other. Synergy takes place from their coupling, creating a stronger, more powerful kind of wave. A standing or stationary wave. The human bio-field is revitalised when exposed to Scalar energy as Scalar energy resonates with the body's healing frequencies.

At least one laser manufacturer combines cold laser technology with Scalar waves.

SOLITON WAVES

Discovered in 1834 by John Scott Russell, **Soliton** is a single, nonlinear wave – actually, it is half a wave, either the crest or the trough. When two of these solitary waves meet, they form a 'soliton wave' that can travel for a long distance whilst retaining their (pre-collision) identity, speed and shape. Solitons occur naturally in nature as tsunamis and the sound waves in water that enable whales and dolphins to communicate. In living matter, a soliton can capture a natural charge and carry it along without requiring further input of energy. The remarkable characteristics of the soliton has important implications in the field of energy healing.

According to bio-physicist and cell biologist, James Oschman:

"Solitons resemble nerve impulses in the body.... Various therapists have noted that waves resembling solitons appear from time to time in the body, and seem to have beneficial effects, including the release and/or resolution of traumatic memories."

Dr. Larry Lytle has incorporated soliton wave technology into his cold laser invention, the QLaser:

"The higher amplitude soliton, created by a meeting of two solitary waves, creates a very low energy output, which harmonizes (resonates) with the human body's energy... [the energy travels] deeply into the body without changing or losing its waveform or the information it carries... Its subtle energy penetrates deeply into all tissues such as ligaments, joints, bones, blood vessels and organs. This energy also carries electrons that re-energize cell membranes damaged by trauma, pollutants, and other forms of stress."

BENEFITS OF SCALAR and SOLITON WAVE

Reduces pain and inflammation

Swelling usually accompanies disease and injury. This is due to a combination of blood and lymph fluids stagnating, and red and white cells clumping together. The Scalar and Soliton wave works both in the field surrounding the body, as well as permeating the body's tissues. It brings about relaxation and dilation of the peripheral blood vessels, and unclumping of the cells. This enhances circulation to enable oxygen-rich blood to be delivered to injured tissue to speed up the body's natural recovery process.

Immune Function

The waves enhance the capabilities of both the immune and endocrine systems to destroy viruses and bacteria. The immune function is purported to be strengthened by up to 149%(!).

Cellular Nutrition and Detoxification

As a result of the unclumping of cells and the enhanced circulation that follows, fluid is able to flow rapidly to deliver nutrients to, and carry waste away from, the cells.

The permeability of cell walls is improved, facilitating the intake of nutrients and the elimination of toxins.

Anti-aging

The aging process is usually accompanied by a decrease in cellular energy levels. Exhaustion, loss of libido, susceptibility to age-related diseases, are some of the symptoms of the slowing-down process. A decrease of cellular energy means that the structured and organised removal of abnormal cells is compromised. This can lead to inflammatory and degenerative diseases. The effect of Scalar and Soliton waves is to restore energy function, energizing the cells to a healthy 70-90 mini volts, thereby de-accelerating the aging process.

DNA

Spectographs have shown Scalar and Soliton energy strengthening the chemical (hydrogen) bonds within DNA, making it resistant to damage and preventing the growth of cancer cells. When these bonds are damaged, some of the DNA's particles break and become cancer cells.

Nervous System

Our brain and nervous system is constantly being bombarded by the negative effects of electro-magnetic stress (EMFs) from computers, phones, microwaves, alarm systems, electric blankets, etc. This leads to a disturbance of the body's homeostasis. Scalar and soliton waves provide a protective shield that cancels the effects of these manmade frequencies (60hz); as well as promoting alpha wave brain frequencies that induce coherence, relaxation, creativity, focus and improved clarity.

As I've already stated, I speak as an independent user. I admit to not being a scientist, and I certainly don't claim to wholly understand the quantum technology of these lasers in the detailed way in which a scientist or physicist would. Nor am I always clear about the impressive, sometimes incomprehensible, declarations of some cold laser developers and distributors. However, by the same token, I couldn't fully describe to you the inner workings of my microwave oven, my personal computer or even the light switches around my home. But I trust the technologies enough to use them daily. This trust is based entirely on my expectations of use; as well as the *results* I achieve from use that assure me that these devices are fit for their intended purpose. Likewise, my own personal experience and the countless (written and visual) testimonials given by laser users speak loudly and evidently for themselves, and simply have to be credited. After all, does one trust the theory and marketing proclamations of a given product, or personal, intuitive and experiential evidence? I know what I opt for, each and every time.

CHAPTER 6
THE BODY SYSTEMS

THE HEALING GATEWAYS

There have been many occasions when, after a healing session, I have been asked by dazed clients whether they had been subjected to hypnotherapy. They ask me this after emerging from a deep and 'zoned-out' sleep that they had slipped into mere seconds or minutes after I placed my hands near their body and directed healing energy into their aura. I explain that what they have just experienced is their body reacting to energy. It is an illusion to think that the healer is responsible for another person's 'healing.' Healing is always an inside job. In the deep, soundless place into which my clients dissolve, it is the infinite intelligence of their own cells performing the healing work of repair and regeneration. Rather than the result of hypnotherapy, my clients are, quite literally, floating in the quantum ocean of *zero-point*.

SIMPLY PUT

Zero-point . The space between the breath. The thought. The emotion. The point at which your mind goes inside and reaches peace and stillness.

Zero-point. Stillpoint. Still Field. The Gap. Neutral Point. These are all attempts to describe that point of silence and motionlessness from which all life and consciousness arises. Think of periods in your life when you became lost in, yet totally a part of, the moment. You listened to a piece of beautiful, captivating music. You held the preciousness of a new-born baby. You looked into the innocent eyes of a trusting and adorable animal. You walked along the beach, admiring the glorious sunset. You gazed at spectacular views from the top of a mountain. At the point of 'no thought,' you were connected to *zero-point*. Zero-point is Equanimity. At this point we are resonating with our Highest Essence. We are witnessing without feelings or emotions, detached from the outcome of the next moment. At the highest level there is

Bliss: the state where you are resonating with unbounded happiness and unconditional love.

This powerful point is the gateway through which we access rejuvenation, healing and manifestation. The amazing thing about your laser is that it can lead you to and through this gateway. By unwinding stress or *cellular memory* (more of this later) from certain vital glands and nerves, your body is able to slip into a state of preparedness for healing. The important areas to direct your laser are the adrenal glands, the sacrum, the cranium, and the thymus.

Hold the Laser against each of the following points for 2-4 minutes, or whatever feels right for you. You will know you are descending into *zero-point* when you begin to experience the signs of varying degrees of relaxation: sighing, yawning, feelings of calm, 'letting go,' stillness, nothingness, expansiveness, boundlessness, centredness, peace, etc.

Following this procedure before any type of session with the laser, allows the body to 'open up' to healing.

HEALING GATEWAYS

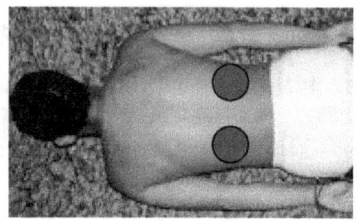

Adrenals

(both left and right adrenals)

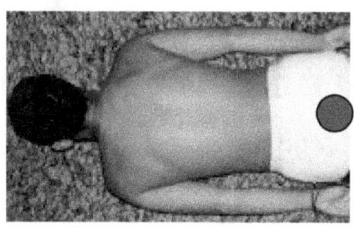

Sacrum

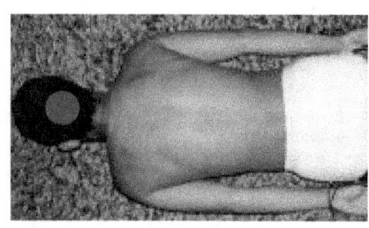

Cranial

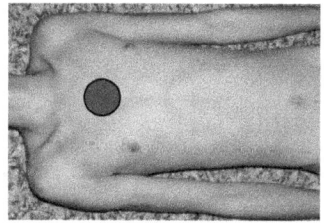

Thymus

❖ **Adrenals** *(Either side of the lower back, above each kidney)*

Adrenal exhaustion is caused by stress – mental, physical, emotional or environmental. When the adrenals are constantly pumping out adrenaline, cortisol and other stress hormones, this can lead to chronic fatigue, changes in blood pressure, depression, recurring infections, reduced sex drive, brain fog, fibromyalgia, hypoglycemia and insomnia.

❖ **Sacrum**   (*Lower spine, coccyx*)

This opens up the nerve pathways down into the legs, stimulating energy flow, bringing blood and oxygen. Pain and inflammation dissolve as new cells start growing. Sacral nerve damage can lead to sciatica as well as bladder and bowel control problems.

❖ **Cranial**   (*Nexus at top of spine/base of the head*
          - occipital ridge)

Protects the vagus nerve, the longest, most complex cranial nerve, extending all the way down into the abdomen. Stimulating this nerve can bring relief from fainting, epilepsy, depression, digestion, swallowing and speech difficulty.

❖ **Thymus**   *(Centre of upper chest)*

When the immune response of the thymus gland is dysfunctional, auto-immune diseases (the body's immune cells reacting against normal body tissues) can occur. These include MS, arthritis, lupus and diabetes.

GLANDS

PINEAL

PITUITARY

THYROID

THYMUS

ADRENAL

PANCREAS

SEXUAL

PROSTATE

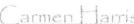

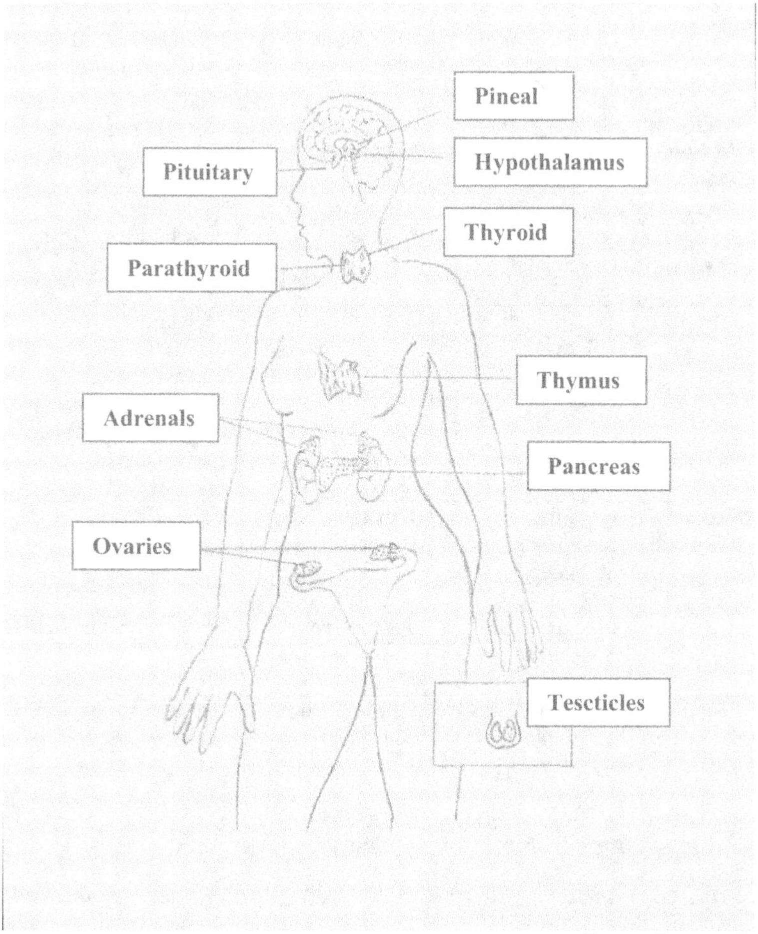

Pineal

Pituitary

Hypothalamus

Thyroid

Parathyroid

Thymus

Adrenals

Pancreas

Ovaries

Tescticles

Rupert Townsend

Glands are organs that produce and/or release substances into
the body, its external surface and the bloodstream. These
hormonal substances regulate growth, metabolism, sexual
development and function.

GLAND	LOCATED	SECRETION	INFLUENCES
Pineal	Centre of brain – 'third eye'	**Melatonin**	Daily biological cycles, including sleep
Pituitary 'Master Gland'	Base of brain	**Numerous hormones**	Growth; Regulation of other endocrine glands
Thyroid	Below Adam's apple	**Thyroxin Calcitonin**	Body heat; Bone growth; Metabolism
Thymus	Chest cavity, behind sternum	**Thymosin**	Immune system
Adrenal	Top of each kidney	**Adrenalin Noradrenalin Corticosteriods**	Metabolism; Blood chemicals; Body characteristics; Nervous system (stress response)
Pancreas	Deep in upper abdomen	**Insulin**	Body's use of glucose
Sexual (Gonads)	(Ovaries - female) Lower abdomen – either side	**Estrogen Progesterone**	Female characteristics
	(Testes - male) Suspended in scrotum	**Testosterone**	Male characteristics
Prostate	Between bladder and penis	**Seminal Fluid**	Semen

Addressing *pineal* and *pituitary* issues: Aim the beam of your infrared pen-laser or probe onto the tip of the nose (avoid looking at the light). This is a direct pathway to the pineal and pituitary glands.

NB: Descartes, French philosopher, mathematician, scientist, and writer, called the pineal gland the 'Seat of the Soul.' This gland (activated by light) is considered to be linked to increased psychic awareness and the highest source of ethereal energy. It is said that when the pineal gland or 'third eye' is awakened, one's frequency is raised, moving one into a higher consciousness.

ORGAN SYSTEMS

BLADDER

BRAIN

COLON

ENDOCRINE SYSTEM

GALLBLADDER

HEART

IMMUNE SYSTEM

KIDNEYS

LIVER

LUNGS

LYMPH SYSTEM

NERVE SYSTEM

PANCREAS

SEXUAL

SKIN

SMALL INTESTINES

SPLEEN

STOMACH

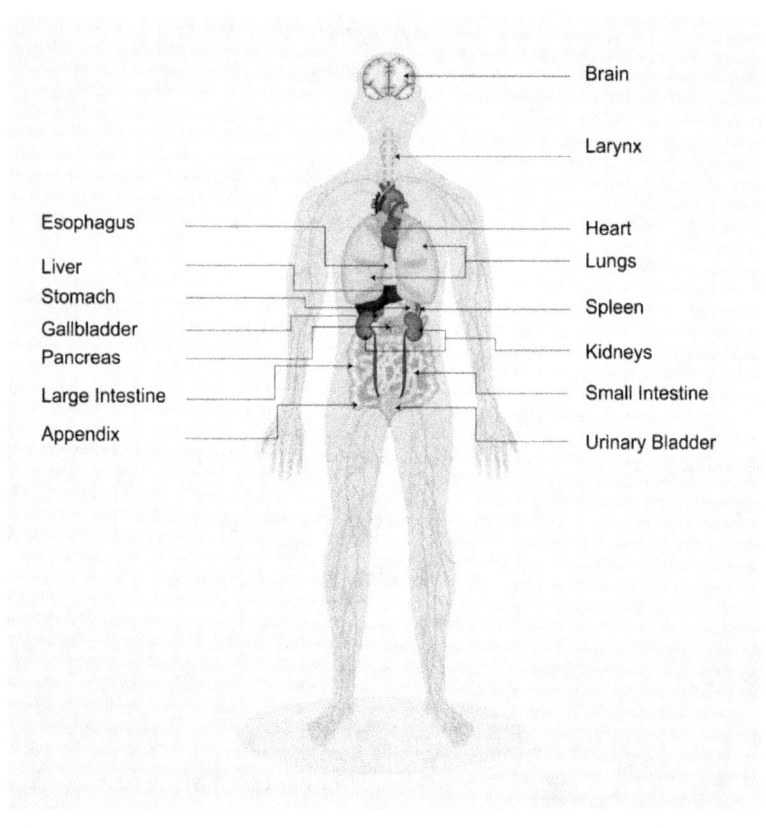

Esophagus
Liver
Stomach
Gallbladder
Pancreas
Large Intestine
Appendix

Brain
Larynx
Heart
Lungs
Spleen
Kidneys
Small Intestine
Urinary Bladder

Stockshoppe 123RF.COM

ORGAN	MAJOR FUNCTIONS	SYMPTOM CHECKER
Bladder	o Temporarily retain urine until it can be released to the urethra and out of the body	o Urgency/frequency urination o Pain/burning with urination o Incontinence o Blood in urine o Cloudy/foul-smelling urine o Pelvic discomfort o Fever o Weight loss o Anaemia
Brain	o Site of consciousness, thought and creativity o Control the body's electrical impulses o Monitor and regulate unconscious processes like heart rate and breathing o Co-ordinate most voluntary movement o Left side controls right side of the body, and vice versa	o Loss of vision / double vision o Eye pain o Dilated pupils o Neck stiffness o Headaches, migraine o Sensitivity to light o Confusion / Memory loss o Ringing in the ears o Nausea, vomiting o Incoherent speech o Behavioural/personality changes o Muscle twitching o Spasms o Seizures o Inability to wake o Muscle weakness on one side o Paralysis
Colon	o Absorption of water and minerals o Formation / elimination of faeces o Contains micro-flora ('friendly' bacteria) to aid digestion, nutrient production, PH (acid-based)	o Constipation – hard, pellet-like stools o Diarrhoea – watery stools o Straining on the toilet o Feeling incomplete after emptying bowels o Blood in stools o Bloating

	balance, and prevent proliferation of harmful bacteria	o Abdominal pain, cramping o Appetite loss, nausea o Fever
Endocrine System	o Regulate slow body processes – mood, growth, tissue, metabolism, sexual function, reproductive processes o Influence every cell, organ, function o Glands involved: hypothalamus, pituitary, thyroid, parathyroid, adrenal, pineal, reproductive	o Specific symptoms depend on the specific part of endocrine affected: Mood / weight / thirst / hunger / fatigue / bladder / bowels / nausea & vomiting / vision changes / overgrowth hands, feet, lips, nose, tongue / joints / headaches / overgrowth bone & cartilage/ skin / libido / sleep / blood sugar / blood glucose / salt cravings / menstruation / bruising / 'moon face' / eyes / throat / breathing / depression / anxiety
Gallbladder	o Aid fat digestion o Stores and excretes bile produced by the liver	o Pain/tenderness under rib cage, right side o Pain between shoulder blades o Jaundice (skin and eyes) o Light or chalky coloured stools o Fatty stools o Indigestion after eating – especially fatty/greasy foods o Nausea o Dizziness o Bloating o Gas, burping or belching o Feeling of fullness, food not digesting o Diarrhoea (soft to watery) o Constipation

		o Headaches over eyes o Bile comes up after eating (biliary)
Heart	o Pump oxygenated blood through the arteries to every cell in the body o Left side receives oxygenated blood from the lungs, circulating it to the tissues o Right side receives de-oxygenated blood from body tissues, sending it to the lungs	o Shortness of breath o Palpitations / irregular heartbeats o Rapid heartbeat o Weakness or dizziness o Nausea o Sweating o Fullness, indigestion, choking feeling o Pressure/heaviness/pain in chest, arm or below breastbone o Discomfort radiating to the back, jaw, throat or arm o Cough, producing white sputum o Swelling in ankles, legs and abdomen o Low grade fever
Immune System	o Identify pathogens (bacteria, parasites, fungus) and tumour cells o Eliminate these from the body – and remember them o White blood cells produced and stored in bone marrow, thymus, spleen, lymph nodes	o Swollen lymph nodes o Frequent serious infections o Persistent or recurrent infections o Infections that don't respond to treatment o Fever, chills o Weight loss o Chronic sinusitis or bronchitis o Growth problems in children
Kidneys	o Remove water and waste from the body o Balance chemicals in the body o Release hormones o Help control blood pressure o Help produce red	o Urinating more or less often o Fatigue o Back pain o Appetite loss, nausea, vomiting o Swelling in hands or feet

	o Produce Vitamin D – for healthy bones blood cells	o Itchiness or numbness o Drowsiness o Lack of concentration o Darkened skin o Muscle cramps
Liver	o Aid digestion o Extract nutrients o Break down harmful drugs, poisons, including alcohol o Store iron, sugars, vitamins and minerals o Regulate fat metabolism and distribution o Produce/maintain balance of hormones o Produce enzymes for the body's chemical reactions – eg tissue repair, blood clotting	o Jaundice o Fever / shivers o Vomiting blood o Fatigue, weakness, poor health o Appetite loss, nausea, vomiting o Weight loss o Abdominal pain/discomfort/ swelling o Itchiness o Tenderness below right ribs o Dark urine o Pale grey or dark tarry stools o Loss of sex drive
Lungs	o Supply oxygen (energy) to the body through nose and mouth o Remove carbon dioxide (waste product) from the body o Produce mucous to defend against infection	o Trouble breathing o Shortness of breath o Hoarseness or wheezing o Persistent cough o Chest tightness o Feeling like you're not getting enough air o Decreased ability to exercise o Coughing up blood or mucous o Pain or discomfort when breathing
Lymph System*	o Drain excess fluid from the tissues o Store white blood cells in lymph nodes to fight infection o Transport protein and large fats from small	o Upper respiratory infection (runny nose, sore throat, fever) o Tender nodes just under skin around ears, under chin, upper part of neck o Enlarged node tracking

	intestines to the blood	towards heart o Skin infection or redness o Chronic cough o Swollen limb
Nerve System	o Sensory neurons – detect and monitor internal and external stimuli o Inter-neurons – transfer, interpret and synthesise signals to create sensations, thoughts, memory o Motor-neurons – sends impulses/signals to muscles and glands to act accordingly	o Confusion o Memory loss o Altered behaviour o Babbling speech o Decreased alertness o Muscle weakness / body fatigue o Headaches o Changes in vision o Dizziness o Lightheadedness o Vertigo o Seizure
Pancreas	o Help break down protein, carbohydrates and fats for body's fuel o Secrete hormones: insulin lowers blood sugar; glucagons raises blood sugar o Neutralise acids that pass from the stomach into small intestines	o Severe abdominal pain o Tender, swollen abdomen o Nausea o Vomiting o Fever, sweating o Rapid pulse o Jaundice o Weight loss o Diabetes

Sexual	o Produce, secrete male sex hormones o Male: Produce, maintain, transport sperm and semen o Discharge sperm in female reproductive tract o Female: Produce egg cells o Receive penis and semen o Transport eggs to site of fertilisation o Development embryo	o Male: urinary frequency, difficulty starting and stopping / inability to empty bladder / pain / burning / fever / chills, pain between scrotum-rectum / fatigue / blood or pus in urine / lower back pain / impotence /premature ejaculation o Female: Abnormal bleeding, spotting / vaginal discharge / burning, itching, stinging, throbbing, numbness / missed periods / pain during intercourse, urination problems / abdominal pain / fatigue / fever and chills / loss appetite
Skin	o Protection – acts as barrier against impacts, pressure, temperature changes, micro-organisms, radiation, chemicals o Regulation – temperature, peripheral circulation, fluid balance (through sweat); reservoir for synthesis of Vit D o Sensation – nerve cell receptors for heat, cold, touch, pain o Excretion – water, urea, ammonia, uric acid	o Bleeding o Bruising o Blisters, cysts, pustules o Bumps, pimples o Burning o Blackheads, whiteheads o Discolouration, change of colour o Dry, cracking, chafing o Fever o Hot, cold, clammy, pale o Impetigo o Inflammation o Moles, warts o Numbness o Pain o Rashes o Scales, flaking o Sensitivity o Sores o Tenderness o Thickening, swelling

Small Intestines	o Digestion of food o Absorption of nutrients and minerals found in food	o Stomach pain, cramps o Nausea, vomiting o Abdominal tenderness/swelling o Appetite loss o Weight loss o Constipation, diarrhoea o Skin condition, acne o Fatigue o Malnutrition
Spleen	o Filter and remove old/ damaged red blood cells o Help produce white blood cells o Store fresh reserves red blood cells o Remove certain harmful bacteria	o Pain upper left abdomen o Pain upper left back or shoulder o Feeling fullness near stomach o Difficulty eating a large meal o Repeated infections o Anaemia o Fatigue o Dizziness o Hiccups
Stomach	o Store the food we eat o Liquidise food into chyme o Create enzymes to break down food o Empties into small intestines	o Burning in throat o Constipation o Diarrhoea o Gas and flatulence o Indigestion o Nausea o Reflux o Vomiting

* Lymph glands are located around the shoulder area, clavicle, stomach area, colon, groin, sides, hips and under arms.

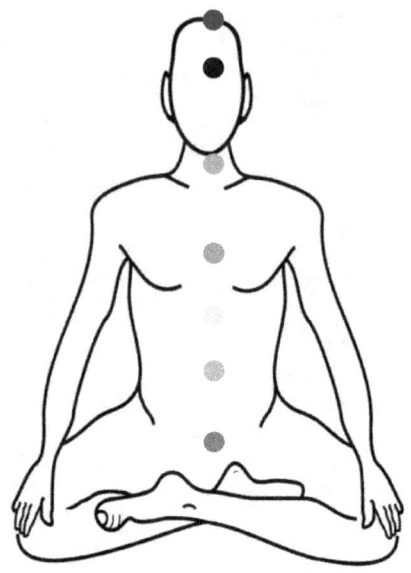

Hana Sarova 123RF.COM

Crown

Third Eye

Throat

Heart

Solar Plexus

Sacral

Root

CHAKRAS

ROOT

SACRAL

SOLAR PLEXUS

HEART

THROAT

THIRD EYE

CROWN

The chakras are energy centres that circulate the flow of energy from the Universe into our body. They are likened to spinning wheels, enabling a two-way flow of Universal energy to activate the body systems. The difference between a corpse and a living being, is this flow of energy. We are three-dimensional beings, yet the chakras exist in the fourth dimension. This means, for most of us the chakras are not accessible to the five senses. However, they do exist, and they play a vital role in both our physical and our emotional health. An imbalance in the flow of energy usually shows up in the auric field (where the chakras reside) before it manifests in the physical body as dis-ease. Each chakra relates to our emotions and to certain parts of the body, in particular the glands and major organs. A disruption in the flow of energy to the chakras will affect its corresponding area. There are many chakras all over the body, seven of which are considered major:

CHAKRA	LOCATION	GLANDS / ORGANS	FEAR OF...
Root	Genitals to tail-bone	*Adrenals*, Rectum, colon, bones, spinal column, hips, legs, feet, large intestines, blood vessels, immune system, nose.	- Change - Rejection
Sacral	Below navel, lower abdomen	*Gonads (ovaries/testes)*, Sexual and reproductive organs, colon, lower back, appendix, bladder, kidneys, hips, sacrum, lower back.	- Losing control - Sensuality
Solar Plexus	Below breastbone, above navel	*Pancreas*, stomach, small intestines, liver, gallbladder, kidneys, spleen, middle spine, upper intestines, lower back, the skin, muscular system, face.	- Not being worthy - Not being loveable - Criticism
Heart	Centre of chest	*Thymus*, lungs, heart, circulatory system, upper chest, upper back, hands, arms.	- Commitment - Betrayal - Loneliness - Vulnerability - Following your heart
Throat	Throat area	*Thyroid*, throat, neck, shoulder, arms. hands, ears, osepophagus, mouth, jaws, teeth, ears, gums, parathyroid, trachea, hypothalamus.	- Speaking your truth - Hurting others
Third Eye	Between eyes	*Pituitary*, brain, left eye, ears, nose, sinus, nervous system.	- Total surrender - Intuition
Crown	Top of head	*Pineal* gland, brain, muscular system, right eye, skeletal system, nervous system, skin.	- Loss of focus - Trusting life

Tip: The chakras exist in the fourth dimension. Experiment by placing your laser several inches off the body so that it is operating in the auric (energy) field.

MERIDIANS

BLADDER
GALLBLADDER
HEART
KIDNEY
LARGE INTESTINES
LIVER
LUNGS
SMALL INTESTINE
SPLEEN
STOMACH

GOVERNOR
CONCEPTION
CONSTRICTOR
ENDOCRINE

The meridians, a network of invisible pathways, travel deep inside the body. Along these meridians, below the skin's surface, there are over 500 acupuncture points. Each meridian is linked to the major organ or system that it services (refer to the section on *Organ Systems* for a general explanation of the location of particular organs).

The meridians carry life-energy ('chi,' 'qi,' 'prana') from the chakras and distribute its flow to energise and nourish the body's tissues and vital organs. When this flow is disrupted, either due to a deficiency or an excess of energy, vulnerability to physical and emotional imbalance can occur.

NB: In place of acupuncture needles, cold lasers are sometimes used to stimulate the body's acupoints. Russian researchers at the Institute for Clinical and Experimental Medicine have shown that light applied to the human skin penetrates the body between 2 and 30 mm. Depending on the colour frequency, certain areas of the body are able to transfer light beneath the surface. These areas correspond to acupuncture points, conducting along the acupuncture meridians. From this research, it appears that the meridians are like optical fibres, transferring light within the body.

The Organ meridian pathways run on both sides, left and right, of the body.

MERIDIAN	PATHWAY	EMOTIONS	IMBALANCE
Bladder	Begin corner of eye, continue over head, down the spine, around buttock cheek, down centre back of thighs and legs, cross at ankle, end on small toe.	Feeling 'pissed off,' inability to express emotions (eg. bed wetting in children), fear, lack of confidence, nervousness, fear of being overwhelmed, strained nerves, lethargy, hypersensitivity	Tension/pain along spine or waist, neurological disorders, low sexual energy, diaorrhoea, night-time incontinence, headaches on defecation, abdominal congestion, cloudy urine, problems with sense of smell, nosebleeds.
Gallbladder	Begin outside of eye, around ear, up and forward over head, double back, travel down to shoulder, down side rib cage, forward onto rib cage, back on the waist, forward on hip, straight down outside of leg, end on fourth toe.	Resentment, timidity, irritability, bitterness, constant sadness, indecisiveness, easily discouraged.	Tension headache, neck/ shoulder pain, insomnia, chest/side pains, leg muscle/tendon weakness; chills, tiredness, bitter taste, joint pain, edema in legs and knees.
Heart	Begin under armpit, down inside arm, side of hand, ends inside little finger.	The heart rules all emotions: Psychological problems, hysteria, erratic behaviour, alternating joy and melancholy, dullness, yearning for love, jealousy, sorrow, nightmares	Heartburn, stuttering, cold feeling in chest/limbs, palpitations, night sweats, memory failure, restless sleep, insomnia, numb/heavy tongue, heavy chest, orange coloured urine.
Kidney	Begin centre of sole of foot, travel up inside leg, up	Poor willpower, fear, guilt, no zest for life,	Immune deficiency, anaemia, lumbago, sciatica, cold feet and

	midline, _end_ collarbone.	nervousness, lack of confidence, depression, trembling, paranoia, loneliness, insecurity, unable to confront situations, low vitality, poor memory, inability to think clearly.	legs, excessive sweating, musculo-skeletal irritation and inflammation, sexual impotence.
Large Intestines	_Begin_ index finger, up arm to shoulder and neck, cross to beneath nose, _end_ on outer edge of nose.	Holding on, not being able to let go of the past, sorrow, resentment, worry, anguish, claustrophobia, inflexibility (emotionally/physically), pessimism, nostalgia, stubbornness.	Constipation, diarrhoea, bloating, colon cancer, skin cancer, TMJ, carpal tunnel syndrome, eczema, psoriasis, chronic rashes, toothaches, sore throat, problems with neck and shoulders.
Liver	_Begin_ inside corner big toe, across to ankle, up inner leg, cross to above waist, up to torso, across, _end_ few inches below nipple.	Anger, irritability, impatience, short temper, hatred, jealousy, power-hungry, over-ambitious, controlling, need to be right (even when wrong), moodiness.	Throat lump, difficulty swallowing, bitter taste, tooth issues, abdominal tension, lumbar pain, muscle/tendon tension lower extremities, insomnia, illnesses of breast and genitals, para/thyroid disturbance, gallbladder/bile duct issues; periodontitis, neuralgia, skin disorders, insomnia, red/watery eyes.
Lungs	_Begin_ on thumb, travel along inside arm, up over shoulder, down and _end_ above nipple,	Grieving, isolation, disconnected from the world, sorrow,	Shallow breathing, lung congestion, pneumonia, bronchitis, asthma, colds, flu, pallid skin,

	inside edge front of shoulder.	resentment, worry, anguish, claustrophobia, inflexibility (emotionally/ph ysically), pessimism, nostalgia.	poor complexion, clogged/runny nose, chest pains.
Small Intestine	Begin end of little finger, up inside arm, cross at elbow, up over shoulder, halfway down shoulder blade, up to side of neck, over to cheekbone, back to ear end in front of ear.	Hearing difficulties, inability to sort out sounds, unclear thoughts, forgetfulness, indecision, restlessness, digestive problems, difficulty expressing emotions.	Food allergies, TMJ, strokes, earache, shoulder/arm/neck pain, difficulty sorting sounds, tinnitus, pain around the ear, abdominal pain.
Spleen	Begin big toe, up inside leg, cross at knee to centre of thigh, up torso in line with nipple, armpit, end midway down ribs on side of body.	Brain fog, scatterbrained, worry, poor concentration, forgetfulness, vacillation, addiction, attachment, obsession, gluttony, jealousy, self-pity, strong concern about opinion of others, stubborn, vain.	Weak limbs, muscular atrophy, morning fatigue, cold/wet feet, taut/distended abdomen, sweet cravings, flatulence, nausea, mild edema, heavy feeling in legs, pale lips, loose stools.
Stomach	Begin under eye, down to jaw, up and around side of face, through side of eye go down face and neck to throat, cross to shoulder blade, down through nipple, in at waist, out to hip, straight down leg, end on second toe.	Being unable to 'stomach' someone or something, worry, nervousness ('butterflies'), anxiety, worry, scepticism, lack of confidence, suspicion, distrust.	Nausea, reflux, eating disorders, ulcers, sinus problems, frontal headache, TMJ, mild rashes.

Below, are the four 'non-Organ' Meridians. (Endocrine and Constrictor pathways run on both sides, left and right, of the body).

MERIDIAN	PATHWAY	FUNCTION	EMOTIONS
Governor	Begins at tailbone, moves up spine, up to neck, over centre of cranium, down centre of forehead and nose, ends upper lip.	Relates to **Masculine** energy and the **Nervous system**. Regulates the functions of the brain, spine marrow, urinary and reproductive systems.	When unbalanced the there is lack of willpower, stubbornness, fatigue, deep coldness, indifference, feeling unsupported and vulnerable to addictions. Deep coldness, chronic urinary/reproductive issues. Stiffness at the nape of the neck can occur. When flowing, you have the 'spine' to deal with life from the strength of your own integrity.
Conception	Begins between anus and genitals, move up centre line of torso, neck, chin, ends below lower lip.	Relates to **Feminine** energy and the **Brain**. Regulates the menstrual flow, reproductive system and the foetus. Regulates chi circulation of the chest, promotes the function of the spleen and stomach.	When unbalanced there is a tendency to depression, mania, obsessions, perfectionism, anxiety, workaholism and feeling unable to meet challenges. Chronic bowel problems; digestion, lung and heart issues; uterine bleeding; infertility. Abnormal masses (eg. hernia in men; enlarged spleen in women) can occur. When flowing, life force and vitality are restored.

Constrictor (Pericardium / Circulation-sex)	Begins just above nipple, goes up chest towards shoulder, along inside arm, through centre of palm, ends at middle finger.	Relates to **Circulation** and **Hormones**. The pericardium is the protective sac around the heart. Excess chi is drawn off by this meridian and disseminated through the energy point in the palm of the hands. Considered to have a direct bearing on sexual energy.	When unbalanced there is insecurity, sorrow, sadness, defensiveness, despairing, gloom, jealousy, hysteria, stubbornness, hyper-sensitivity, sleeplessness, general feelings of defencelessness and surrendering easily to illness. Pain in the heart area, poor circulation, stomach issues. When flowing, life-force circulates joyfulness, playfulness and creativity.
Endocrine (Triple Warmer)	Begins at ring finger, follows outer arm, up to shoulder, up to neck, around ears, through temples, ends outer edge of eyebrow.	Relates to the **Thyroid, Adrenals, Temperature Control, Immune** and **Survival Responses**. Three sections relate to the upper body (including head), middle body, and lower abdomen. Produces heat in the body and helps regulate fluid balance.	When unbalanced there is a tendency towards hopelessness, panic, isolation, forgetfulness, rambling thoughts, hysteria, burnouts, poor reasoning, laziness and lack of communication and focus. Imbalance can manifest as deafness, tinnitus, bloating, edema, urinary difficulties, fever, shivers, sore throat, headaches. When flowing, metabolism is regulated and mental, physical and emotional energy are in balance.

There are many diagrammatic books and online references on the subject of meridians.

Experiment using your laser probe to trace the pathway of particular meridians.

CELLULAR

BLOOD
BONES
CAPILLARIES
CELL REGENERATION
DISC
DNA
EARS
FACIAL
FASCIA
FAT CELLS
LIGAMENTS
MUSCLES
NEURONS
RNA
SCAR

CELLULAR MEMORY

Dr Deepak Chopra
(Quantum Healing)

Dr Chopra describes the concept of suppressed negative emotions - stress and trauma - being stored as 'cellular or phantom memories' in cells throughout our body. These cellular memories influence us energetically/vibrationally over time, eventually causing emotional and physical illness.

The body is composed of trillions of cells, the elementary unit of all life. As old cells die, new cells are born to replace them. This process of biochemical activity repeats itself every nano-second of our lives. Eye cells take only 48 hours to completely regenerate and form a new eye. The liver totally renews in 6 weeks.

Question: If our bodies are programmed to regenerate in this way, why is it that diseased cells are not always replaced with healthy cells?

Answer: When trauma and negative emotions are unresolved, they manifest physically as cellular memory. Instead of passing on the memory (blueprint) of health, the cells pass on the old 'stuck' programmes of dis-ease: old emotions, old memories, old stresses, old injuries, years after the original trauma occurred.

Your laser's technology helps the cells to dissolve and release these memories so that healing can take place and the body is restored as a coherent system of communication and organisation.

Below are descriptions of the various cellular systems. Use your laser to bring more energy to the injury/contracted site, to shift polarities and transform issues.

CELLULAR SYSTEMS

Blood	Transport system of the body. Red and white blood cells and molecules carry water, oxygen, carbon dioxide, food, waste and chemical messages around the body. White blood cells defend against infection.
Bones	We have 206 bones, dense, white tissue composing the skeleton. Their function is to support and give shape to the body; protect the brain, spinal cord and vital organs; and produce blood cells and store minerals. The largest bone in the body is the femur; the smallest can be found in the ear.
Capillaries	Smallest blood vessel in the body - the walls are one cell layer thick - passing blood from the arteries to the veins. Broken capillaries (rosacea) can be seen on the surface of the skin. As the skin ages and thins, these capillaries can become more prominent. Alcoholism can worsen the condition.
Cell Regeneration	Normal, healthy cells regenerate, passing on the blueprint for the next generation of healthy cells – unless cellular memory inhibits this process. Neuroscientists have recently discovered that, contrary to previous opinion, the brain can repair itself and grow new cells.
Disc	Act as shock absorbers between the vertebrae. They are also like a ligament holding the vertebrae of the spine together. Each disc is like a jelly doughnut with a tough outer part and a soft inner core. There are 23 vertebrae and problems with these can cause back pain, neck pain and sciatica.
DNA	Molecules found in all living things. Can be likened to the computer that houses the programming code (genetic instructions) for individual cells to function and develop.

Ears	Composed of three parts. The *Outer* ear collects sound signals; the *Middle* ear contains the ear drum that translates the sound waves into vibrations; in the *Inner* ear these vibrations cause the tiny hairs covering the cochlea to create nerve signals that the brain understands as sound. The inner ear is also responsible for maintaining our balance.
Facial	Our skin acts as a barrier and a filter from the external environment. External stresses (sun, smoking, gravity, facial expressions, etc.) and the normal aging process (biochemical changes affecting Ph balance, collagen, elastin and turnover of skin cells) lead to wrinkles and thin, dry, sagging skin.
Fascia	Arrangement of dense, connective collagen fibres. This flexible tissue is like wrapping which either suspends organs in place; bind structures together (eg. nerves and blood vessels); or permit structures (eg. muscles) to slide smoothly over each other.
Fat cells	Store excess energy from foods as fat. When fat is released, the cells shrink. Fat cells also act as an insulator and provide protective cushioning.
Ligaments	Band of tough fibrous tissue that keeps the skeletal bones in alignment, connecting the muscles, bone to bone, or bone to cartilage. Ligaments are also sheets of membrane that support muscles or keep an organ in place – eg. part of the liver to the diaphragm and abdominal wall. Ligaments can be stretched (sprain) or torn.
Muscles	There are over 600 muscles both inside (many of them involuntary, like the heart muscle) These have fibrous tissue that has the ability to contract and relax to produce movement. Inside the muscles, nerves carry messages to and from the brain; blood vessels carry the necessary energy and transport waste.

Neurons	Basic building block of the nervous system. These specialised nerve cells transmit information throughout the body – communicating with the brain (sensory), the muscles (motor neurons), and other neurons (inter-neurons). Neurons die but are not replaced. However, new connections between neurons form throughout life.
RNA	Produced by DNA, these molecules transcribe the DNA code so that it can be translated into protein – muscles, bone, blood, body organs.
Scar	Fibrous connective tissue (fibrosis) as a result of wound repair from accident, disease or surgery. Original skin tissue is made of randomised protein (collagen) fibres, but in scar tissue the replacement fibres are aligned in a single direction. This produces inferior tissue lacking sweat glands and hair follicles. Scarring can occur on the skin, the largest organ in the body, or internally (lesions).

ALCHEMIC PROCESSES

**5HTP
ENDORPHINS
ENKEPHALIN
FRONTAL LOBE
HYDROGEN
NEUROMUSCULAR
OZONE
SEROTONIN
SILICA**

We live in an infinite, pulsating quantum ocean of energy that is freely available to all of us. Energy is the real substance behind all matter and form. This energy surrounds us, permeating each one of us, every part of us, and every single thing that exists. When we are free from tension and anxiety, our energies are flowing, rejuvenating and revitalising our cells to optimise our immune function and bring about healing and balance. When we are stressed and exhausted, we lack the ability to optimally process this energy. Common signs of stress include: easily distracted, flustered or overwhelmed, anxiety, panic, prone to being upset, difficulty making decisions, frequent headaches, chest pains, sleep problems, increased smoking and intake of alcohol and/or coffee.

'Alchemy' - the shifting of energies from one state to another. Our body system's natural alchemic processes work through our thoughts, feelings and actions - affecting our baseline for emotional/physical health. Your laser is designed to activate nervous and chemical processes to unwind trauma, circulate the blood and re-organise the body's cells into a vital and communicating system that transforms energy from stagnant and lethargic to flowing and nourishing.

5HTP	Neuro-transmitter that decreases the stress response so that serotonin can be produced.
Endorphins	Naturally produced pain-killers that bring about a natural high, blocking pain signals produced by the nervous system. The blissful feeling one experiences after making love is due to the production of endorphins. As well as relieving pain, endorphins enhance the immune system, reduce stress and delay the aging process.
Enkephalin	Naturally occurring morphine-like substances. While endorphins block pain transmission at the brain stem, enkephalin blocks pain impulse at the spinal cord, restoring well-being and calm.
Frontal Lobe	This part of the brain is involved in motor functions, consciousness, emotions, reasoning, judgment, planning, memory, and impulse control. Frontal lobe settings calm and relax the brain when it is over-taxed in any of these areas. Enhances the communication between left and right hemispheres of the brain. Re-establishes acid/alkaline balance of the tissues.

Hydrogen	Hydrogen is necessary for ATP production. When high amounts of hydrogen are present in the body, fewer acids and free radicals are formed. Helps to detox and balance areas of high alkalinity. Supports diabetics with better cholesterol control, reducing the potential for heart disease and other degenerative disease.
Neuro-muscular	There is a fine balance between the central nervous system (brain, spinal cord, nerves) and the musculo-skeletal system (skeleton and voluntary muscles). When nerve cells become unhealthy or die, communication between the two breaks down. Weakness can lead to twitching, cramps, aches, pains, and joint movement problems.
Ozone	Helps to reduce acidity in the body by oxygenating and detoxing.
Serotonin	Our 'happy hormone.' Neurotransmitters regulate our moods, appetite and sexuality to bring about calm and even wound healing. These feel-good hormones release us from low self-esteem, fear, anxiety, panic, phobias, obsession and pessimism.
Silica	Gives strength and firmness to the body tissues – bones, cartilage, connective tissues, arteries and skin. Strengthens skin, hair, nails, joints and connective tissues. Helps speed up healing of a fracture. Keeps arteries flexible and benefits cardiovascular system.

A WORD ON THE PROBES

Some cold lasers have a main unit with probe attachments that can either be bought separately or as a combination package.

Q: *What is the probe for?*

A: The probes' energy is more direct and focused. It usually emits more energy, coming from a single diode. Probes are good for using on small, or inaccessible areas – eg. a blemish; the ear lobe; the gums, a particular tooth, etc.

Q: What's the difference between probes?

A: **Red**: Visible red light penetrates up to 0.5 inches.

Good for soft to medium tissue, surface cells and soft cells – skin, cartilage right up to the skin, muscle, nerve, meridians, gums, etc.

Infra-red: Laser light penetrates to depth 2-3 inches.

Better for working on medium to hard tissue: teeth, tendon, cartilage, bones, discs, etc.

Below are some popular uses for the probes. Though the main unit can usually be used, the probes have the extra ability to direct energy onto specific points and emit greater energy for a more effective outcome.

Anti-Aging

Use the probe over the entire face, moving it slowly around the area, concentrating on wrinkles and problem areas, to stimulate the firming effects of collagen. Close your eyes and keep the laser's beam away from your eyes.

Weight Loss

Direct the Infra-red probe onto the tip of the nose for several minutes at a time. This is said to activate the metabolism, working with the spleen and thyroid to reduce food cravings and make the body more alkaline. The fat cells beneath the skin begin to emulsify and their leaked contents are naturally expelled from the body. This treatment is usually repeated over a period of a few weeks.

Smoking Cessation

Direct the Infra-red probe on the top central cartilage of the ear. Move the probe slowly around till you have covered the entire ear (excluding the ear canal). The laser's beam is said to stimulate the cells to produce serotonin and endorphins which reduce the cravings that are a result of nicotine withdrawal.

Allergy Relief

Sandi Radomski, naturopathic doctor, writes:

"Acupuncture points on the ear represent all of the other areas of the body. The ear, like the foot and hand, is a hologram of the entire body... [but] has the strongest response. Holding* or thinking about a reactive substance creates an imbalance in the body's energy system... Stimulating the ear points [with your laser, whilst thinking about or holding the substance] will balance the body's energy system in relation to that thought or substance."

*Handle reactive substances with caution. If necessary, seek medical advice.

✳✳✳

CHAPTER 7

ROYAL RIFE & HEALING FREQUENCIES
Unsung Hero: Fact or Hollywood Fiction?

The term *frequency* explains the vibration of energy in all things. Everything is in movement, vibrating at its own unique frequency. All matter and non-matter in the known Universe - every species, every molecule, every thought, every emotion - vibrates or *oscillates* at a particular rate. That includes the moon, the trees, the food you eat, the chair you are sitting on, the page you are turning, and yourself. Every organ, bone, tissue and system in the body is in a state of vibration. Just because we can't see or sense this movement, doesn't mean it isn't happening. On the contrary, this vibration can be detected and measured. As previously mentioned, modern medicine uses frequencies to make diagnoses of structural and pathological disorder: EKG's for the heart; EEG's for the brain; MRI's for damaged cells;

89

PET's for tissue and organ function. When frequencies vibrate in harmony, this is called *resonance*. When frequencies cause imbalance this is called *dissonance*.

The radiation emitted from x-rays has its own frequency that does not resonate with the human frequency – which is why long-term exposure can damage our health. The same applies to the radiation from cell phones. Sometimes ordinarily benign substances can also cause imbalance or dissonance with our own frequency. For example, if you are allergic to strawberries, this is an indication that your frequency is not resonating with the frequency of the strawberry. Whereas, anything that feels healing, soothing, or restorative to the body and mind, is usually an indication that the object or substance is in balance with our frequencies. When our mind and bodies are resonant and in balance, we are vital and healthy.

We can illustrate frequencies by looking at how an intense musical note can shatter a wine glass. You're probably familiar with the cliché of the opera singer demonstrating this. Undetected by the senses, the molecules in the glass are already vibrating at a particular frequency. When the opera singer's volume and musical note matches (resonates with) and exceeds this frequency, the glass shatters. This example is relevant to the story you are about to hear. If this story were not true, you would be excused for thinking that it was Hollywood fiction.

RAYMOND ROYAL RIFE
(1888-1971)

Born in San Diego, Rife was an optical engineer and technician. He was the first person to view a living virus. In the late 1920's he invented a powerful optical microscope, the Universal Microscope, able to magnify objects to 60,000 times their size that enabled far tinier particles to be examined than had ever been possible before. Unlike modern high magnification microscopes that kill the object of its study, for the first time, individual living pathogens - bacteria, viruses and fungi – could be made visible. This was achieved by using a light frequency that matched the pathogen's own resonance frequency, causing it to glow.

Rife discovered that when he intensified the frequencies (in the same way as the volume/musical note for the wine glass), the pathogens exploded. This led to Rife's invention of the Frequency Generator, a device that produced the exact frequencies needed to destroy various viruses. It took Rife many years of painstaking work until he discovered the frequencies which specifically destroyed a vast and impressive number of dangerous disease organisms, including herpes, polio, spinal meningitis, tetanus and influenza. Once he discovered the radio waves of the same light frequency that resonated naturally with each of these microbes, Rife increased or 'spiked' their natural oscillations until they distorted and disintegrated. Incredibly, this 'mortal oscillatory rate' left the surrounding tissue unharmed. So, of Rife's two amazing inventions, one identified and made visible living pathogens; and the other destroyed them by using the specific frequency of a shock wave.

In particular, Rife observed the effect of this procedure on cancer viruses. His world, however, was about to fall apart when he declared that cancer was caused by microbes. He studied how these cancer viruses or microbes changed form according to the environment, how quickly they replicated in response to carcinogens, and how they transformed normal cells into tumour cells. In 1934 at a clinic in California, using Rife technology, 16 advanced stage cancer sufferers were exposed to the same frequencies that would destroy the virus causing their illness. The treatment lasted only minutes (repeated over a course of several days), and was 100% effective. What's more, it caused no adverse symptoms in the persons being treated.

Rife's discoveries threatened certain money-making powers of the day. He and his team were attacked by the AMA (American Medical Association) and there followed a series of events that led to a steady annihilation of his work. Rife's components, photographs, films and written records mysteriously disappeared after a series of break-ins. His virus microscopes were also vandalised. Just as scientists at the Burnett Lab in New Jersey were preparing to announce confirmation of Rife's work, an arson fire inexplicably destroyed the building. The only company, Beam Ray, producing Rife's frequency instruments was bankrupted by a frivolous lawsuit taken against it. Doctors who tried to defend Rife lost their grants and hospital privileges. The medical journals refused to publish any paper by anyone on Rife's therapy, and Rife's own research papers were purged from those journals. Later, police illegally confiscated the remainder of Rife's 50 years of research.

Even to this day, the scientific establishment, not familiar with Rife's work, claim that it is generally impossible to see or identify a living virus with any optical microscope. At the age of 83, Rife died from a combination of alcohol and Valium.

So, what does this sad story have to do with cold laser technology? Everything! The particular frequencies of viruses, bacteria, disease states, healthy organs, and even thoughts and emotions have been identified – as a direct result of Rife and his intense work. Your laser uses frequencies that match or resonate with numerous conditions or states of the human body. We either want to induce those states (eg. Relaxation, Well-being); enhance the functioning of body systems (eg. Liver, Blood); or transform certain conditions (eg Muscle Cramp, Headache).

SIMPLY PUT

The Laser feeds the cells with photon energy to either support or purge an existing frequency.

The frequencies (or wavelengths) that you select either:

- o Amplify the body's cellular frequencies to a healing or normal state, *or*

- o Disrupt those unwanted frequencies that are causing disharmony or imbalance

The energy waves of your laser carry these frequencies in the same way that wifi, cell phones and radios carry information.

Rife, considered to be the father of frequency medicine, provided the basic building blocks of frequency healing. Other key pioneers in the field that dedicated their lives to these frequencies - and who also faced differing levels of persecution and ostracism - were Dr Albert Abrams, Dr Ruth Drown, Dr Hulda Clark, Paul Nogier and Jack Swartz. Without the remarkable work of Royal Rife, these other researchers and scientists, and Rife's loyal supporters who protected his surviving research, your cold laser might be just a thing of Hollywood science fiction.

PART II

✳✳✳

CHAPTER 8

DESIGN YOUR OWN LASER!

IMPORTANT NOTE

**The reader accepts full responsibility for any
frequency programming.**

No medical claims are intended or implied.

This is where the real fun begins! I was excited enough when
I first got my hands on my very own laser, but the day I
grasped the possibilities of customising my laser to suit my
personal needs, is when I discovered that my enthusiasm
knew no bounds!

Each one of us comes to the knowledge of the cold laser as a
result of an unresolved concern in our lives. That issue is

usually physical (arguably, emotion-based; typically stress-related), and can be anything from bunions to breathing difficulties. Your laser will feature various pre- or auto-programmed frequencies that you can use to address whatever symptoms you wish to relieve.

You may, however, like the idea of supplementing your pre-programmed laser protocols with precise frequencies that apply directly to your particular state or condition. There is, for example, an actual a frequency that relates precisely to Bunions. There are also frequencies specifically for Asthma or even Pleurisy, if these are your medical conditions. There are tens of thousands of different frequencies for different states and conditions that you can use, giving you the power and the freedom to customise your laser to your individual requirements. For example, I've always had an issue with varicose veins on my left leg. I began by using the programmes on my own laser that I guessed would relate to this condition: Blood and Capillaries. When I discovered that there was also a Varicose frequency 'out there,' I happily added that to my therapeutic menu. Why limit yourself?

Using PROGRAMMABLE FEATURES:

o   Enables you to use specific frequencies to target specific conditions

o   Increases your overall options

o   Puts you in control

> *'Hi Carmen, I feel so much better already, as soon as I got home yesterday I went to the toilet and my <u>bloating</u> [and <u>constipation</u>] has stopped too. Thanks so much for your help.'*
> *S.M (Student)*
>
> *'I hope S has been in touch with you. I just wanted to say that she felt so much better as soon as she stepped through the door after seeing you on Tuesday. She's been going to the loo, and has also managed to complete an essay that before she was saying she just couldn't do. So once again you have worked a miracle.' (Mother)*

One of my clients sent her teenage daughter to me because she'd been feeling bloated, constipated and unhappy for several weeks. I used EFT to tap on the girl's issues of anxiety over impending exams, and applied some hands-on healing. I also placed my laser on her abdomen (using Constipation and Colon frequencies – see following sections) for approximately 5 minutes each. At the end of the session she looked considerably happier and lighter. Before she left I jokingly told her that I expected an email telling me that she'd achieved a healthy bowel movement! Mother and daughter sent me separate emails (above).

You may argue that EFT and the hands-on healing made an obvious difference to this girl's condition, and I wouldn't dispute that. However, I later used my laser on those same settings for my own bout of constipation. No EFT. No hands-on healing. The effects were just as satisfactory. I now use these protocols regularly as part of my own health regime and routine maintenance. The result (and this is probably far too much information) is that I have increased my bowel regularity to a super-healthy often-twice daily. Here are two other PROGRAMMABLE / CUSTOM examples:

> My daughter dropped a suitcase weighing 15kg on the back of her hand. It was very painful, and right away she could see blood appearing below the skin's surface. She'd only just bought her laser but had already programmed in a BRUISE frequency from an earlier incident. She could tell, however, that this bruise was going to be ugly. She placed the Laser on her hand during the 45 minute journey to the airport. The next day her hand was completely clear!

> At one of my regular Meetups held at my home, one of the ladies, who was barefooted, was complaining about her ARTHRITIC TOE. I asked her how painful it was and she said 7 (out of 10). I gave her my laser to use on her toe. After about 30 minutes I asked her how she was feeling. She said the pain had gone completely! But she added that when she put her shoes on she was sure it would return, as that was when it was most painful. She put her shoes on and was very surprised as there was still no pain!

Many of the healing frequencies that follow in the next section are original Rife frequencies, and others are frequencies that have latterly been added by researchers and scientists to the existing list. They can all be found on the internet. But to make it easier for you, I have included a large selection in this Handbook.

NB: The case studies in this book are personal anecdotes. They do not constitute medical evidence of healing.

Examples are for information and illustration purposes only. Please take medical advice and use personal discretion when making decisions about your own health.

ABC MINOR AILMENTS

NB: What follows are suggestions only, and not a substitute for professional medical care. If you are worried about any of your symptoms, ALWAYS seek medical advice.

o I have listed over 70 conditions with accompanying **Custom** frequencies. Where there is more than one set of Custom frequencies listed (each set is separated by a double space and ends with ~), sample the first and assess the results before trying the subsequent. There is no problem in trying both concurrently; it is so you can separately evaluate the effects of each set of frequencies.

o Where I have included **Tips**, I have tried to go for the less obvious remedies we are all familiar with. All tips are aimed at speeding up healing and reducing discomfort, and are OK to combine with use of your cold laser.

o Don't forget that you can use your **probes** for specific or hard-to-get-at places – ears, mouth, cuts, blisters, etc. Use Red for skin, soft tissue and surface issues; Infra-red for more dense tissue such as bone and cartilage.

o Regarding how long you should use each setting, trust your **intuition**.

o In all cases, I would recommend beginning each of your sessions by opening your **Healing Gateways** (page 54).

__NB:__ When programming Custom frequencies, they should be the full value after the decimal point. For example: 10 = 10.00; 1.5 = 1.50.

DENTAL ISSUES:

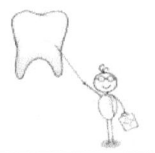

ABSCESS

CUSTOM	2720, 2170, 880, 787, 727, 190, 500 ~ (Staphylococcal infections) 0.05, 0.41, 0.80, 5.25, 87.50, 42.50, 112.33, 375.16, 753.23, 988.90 ~
TIPS	Place dry teabag at site of abscess to draw out toxins. Change as needed; Brush teeth after every meal and rinse with salt water; Fill empty teabag with crushed cloves. Roll into cigar shape. Place on abscess.

DENTAL FOCI, GINGIVITIS, PYORRHEA

CUSTOM	3000, 95, 190, 47.5, 2720, 2489, 1800, 1600, 1550, 802, 1500, 880, 832, 787, 776, 727, 666, 650, 600, 465, 5170, 646 ~
TIPS	The presence of dental foci can affect recovery from ANY illness; Try General Antiseptic frequencies below (Tooth Extraction).

HALITOSIS

CUSTOM	1550, 802, 880, 787, 727, 20 ~
TIPS	Chew basil leaves or fennel after eating food; Drink pineapple juice.

TOOTH EXTRACTION (FOLLOW UP)

CUSTOM	3000, 2720, 95, 47.5, 7.82 ~ (General antiseptic) 10000, 855, 787, 760, 777, 660, 450 ~
TIPS	Try applying cotton wool soaked in clove oil.

EYES, EARS, NOSE, THROAT:

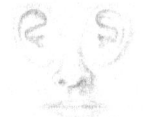

CATARRH

CUSTOM	1550, 802, 800, 880, 787, 727, 444, 20 ~
TIPS	Add raw crushed garlic to your food, or eat straight.

COMMON COLD

CUSTOM	0.12, 0.55, 0.85, 7.50, 120, 247.50, 472.50, 725.75, 850, 975.98 ~ (head/chest) 400, 660, 727, 770, 776, 780, 787, 800, 880 ~
TIPS	Be aware that by the time you feel the symptoms you have already been infected. Try lime juice in warm water, sweetened with honey; Drink chicken noodle soup made with chicken bones.

CONJUNCTIVITIS

CUSTOM	0.17, 0.52, 0.60, 0.85, 225.53, 327.50, 455.95, 760, 850, 969.71 ~
TIPS	Place a raw slice of potato on the affected eye. Repeat for several nights; Treat with drops of rosewater.

COUGHING

CUSTOM	522, 524, 525, 146, 1500, 1550, 0.5, 514, 530, 432, 440, 444, 720, 1234, 3702, 20, 125, 72, 95, 7.7 ~ 0.07, 0.24, 0.91, 7.50, 12.08, 145.50, 442, 574.50, 797.50, 983.50 ~
TIPS	Productive cough – I tsp raw onion juice mixed with 1 tsp honey. Take twice daily. Dry cough – steam inhalation moisturizes dry, irritated passageways; Take frequent sips of water (avoid chilled).

EAR CONDITIONS
(DISCHARGE, TINNITUS, ITCHING, HEARING LOSS)

CUSTOM	9.19, 10000, 880, 787, 727, 20, 410, 158, 201, 340, 440, 535, 542, 645, 652, 683 ~
TIPS	A few drops of fresh breast milk(!) inside the ear is said to be beneficial for ear discharge.

EAR INFECTION (OTITIS)

CUSTOM	0.10, 0.52, 0.78, 0.80, 2.25, 5.26, 167.50, 352.52, 845.47, 922.53 ~ 727, 787, 880, 174, 482, 5311 ~
TIPS	Try swim ear plugs for children if they spend a lot of time in the water; or are using a public pool and susceptible to these infections, Use a blow-dryer at a safe distance away from head to dry out trapped water in inner ear.

EAR WAX

CUSTOM	311, 320, 750, 984 ~
TIPS	If a persistent condition, consider ear candling.

HICCUP

CUSTOM	20, 10000 ~
TIPS	Fill mouth with a tablespoon of sugar, suck slowly; Block both ears and drink 6 ounces of water without stopping to breathe. Hold breath for as long as possible, then let it out.

HOARSENESS

CUSTOM	880, 760, 727 ~
TIPS	Add few drops of lemon and ¼ tsp of cayenne pepper to a cup of warm water. Sip slowly and take throughout the day; Add one tsp apple cider vinegar to half glass water. Take every hour throughout the day; Suck on ice.

RHEUMA
(WATERY NOSE / EYES)

CUSTOM	952, 436, 595, 775 ~
TIPS	Nose – Eat spicy food! Encourages discharge, flushing out what is causing the symptoms; Dissolve ½ tsp salt in glass of warm water and draw some into a dropper. Tilt head back and irrigate nostril. Do this several times, then blow nose. Eyes – Wash eyes in some cooled coriander water (coriander boiled in water); Soak soft cloth in cooled turmeric water (1/2 litre water, 6 gram of turmeric powder, boil till reduced to half), place on eyes.

SINUSITIS

CUSTOM	728, 784, 880, 20, 72, 120, 146, 400, 440, 464, 524, 548, 660, 712, 732, 802, 1500, 1552, 1600, 1862 *for 5 min* ~ 125, 160, 367, 472, 600, 615, 625, 650, 820, 952, 1150, 1520, 1865, 2000, 4392, 4400, 4412 ~ 60, 95, 128, 225, 414, 427, 432, 456, 610, 614, 618, 1234, 2600, 5500, 304 ~ (Frontalis) 952, 320, 682 ~ (Maxillaris) 160, 741 ~
TIPS	Drink 2tbsp apple cider vinegar in 8oz water at first sign of symptoms.

SNEEZING

CUSTOM	880, 787, 727, 465, 146 ~
TIPS	Dissolve ½ tsp salt in glass of warm water and draw some into a dropper. Tilt head back and irrigate nostril. Do this several times, then blow nose.

SORE THROAT

CUSTOM	2720, 2489, 1800, 1600, 1550, 802, 880, 787, 776, 727, 46.5, 766 ~ (Strep infection) 0.15, 0.70, 2.50, 5.25, 47.50, 70, 275, 425.75, 842, 932 ~
TIPS	Inhale vapours of eucalyptus oil; Take 4 garlic cloves mixed with 1tbsp honey and pinch of cayenne pepper, chew thoroughly before swallowing.

STYE

CUSTOM	10000, 880, 787, 727, 20, 453, 2600 ~
TIPS	Try gently rubbing a gold ring (at least 18K) in the area of the stye.

THROAT TICKLE

CUSTOM	120, 666, 690, 727, 787, 800, 880, 1560, 1840, 1998, 766, 776 ~
TIPS	Gargle with warm water and sea salt; Gargle with apple cider vinegar (few tbsp) and warm water; Take Vitamin C.

TINNITUS

CUSTOM	20, 2720, 728, 784, 880 ~
TIPS	Add 1 tsp salt and 1 tsp glycerine to warm water. Spray into nostril to drain into back of throat. Also spray throat. Repeat 3 times day.

TONSILITIS

CUSTOM	1.2, 73, 1550, 802, 1500, 880, 832, 787, 776, 727, 650, 625, 600, 465, 144, 452, 582 ~
TIPS	Gargle with mustard powder dissolved in warm water.

MUSCULO-SKELETAL:

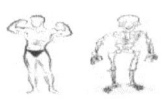

ARTHRITIS

CUSTOM	0.05, 0.75, 0.90, 9.00, 11.09, 55.33, 325.16, 425.71, 642.91, 980 ~
TIPS	If you are non-vegetarian, eat oxtail and bone marrow as regular part of diet; add 4 tbsp Epsom salts to bath water; Sleep with red flannel wrapped around painful joints.

ARTHRITIS (RHEUMATOID)

CUSTOM	0.19, 1.00, 2.80, 17.50, 45, 225, 510.25, 682.02, 759.83, 932.41 ~
TIPS	Include calcium, magnesium and Vitamin C in your diet; Add 4 tsps blackstrap molasses to a quart of cranberry juice, drink one glass daily.

BACKACHE SPASMS

CUSTOM	120, 212, 240, 424, 465, 528, 760, 727, 787, 880, 1550, 2112, 5000, 10000 ~
TIPS	Check whether your diet is sufficient in calcium and potassium; During a spasm, don't forget to BREATHE – slowly and deeply - into the diaphragm. Send your slow out-breath to the area of the spasm.

BACK PAIN (LUMBAGO)

CUSTOM	9.3, 9.4, 9.6, 7.6, 7.7, 3, 0.5, 432, 465, 727, 728, 776, 784, 787 ~ 0.14, 0.40, 7.50, 55, 96.50, 376.29, 425.09, 571, 833, 932 ~ 10000, 800, 880, 787, 727, 125, 95, 72, 444, 1865, 9.19, 8.25, 7.69, 300 ~
TIPS	Massage area with mint oil.

FRACTURES, BONE

CUSTOM	0.13, 0.57, 0.78, 0.93, 32.50, 217.50, 552.71, 743.01, 815.91, 913.52 ~
TIPS	Calcium, Magnesium, and Potassium are essential to repair bone damage.

FROZEN SHOULDER

CUSTOM	10000, 880, 802, 787, 727 ~
TIPS	Every physical ailment/condition has an emotional root. Examine what areas in your life you feel unsupported, unappreciated and overloaded, and what you can do about it.

HIP PAIN

CUSTOM	880, 787, 727, 20 ~
TIPS	Try placing the laser on the hip area as well as the sacrum.

KNEE JOINT PAIN

CUSTOM	1550, 880, 802, 787, 727, 28, 20, 7.69, 3, 1.2, 250, 9.6, 9.39 ~
TIPS	Drink plenty of water daily; Rub joint with hot vinegar before going to bed; Sleep with red flannel wrapped around joint.

MUSCLE CRAMP

CUSTOM	0.13, 0.40, 0.62, 3.83, 35.25, 132.25, 282.50, 327.50, 522.50, 748 ~
TIPS	Use warm towel or heated pad on the affected area; Make sure you are not dehydrated; Take an Epsom salts bath.

MUSCULAR PAIN/INJURY

CUSTOM	2720, 6000, 320, 250, 240, 160, 125, 80, 40, 20, 10, 5.8, 2.5, 1.5, 1.2, 1, 0.5 ~
TIPS	Zinc helps repair tissue damage.

NECK PAIN

CUSTOM	0.08, 0.49, 0.73, 0.80, 7.50, 142.53, 285.02, 412.03, 528.23, 775.56 ~
TIPS	The body uses metaphor to communicate with us. Ask yourself, who or what in my life is a pain in the neck? This will identify what is causing the stress that is leading to neck pain.

SCIATICA

CUSTOM	0.19, 0.50, 0.70, 0.97, 14.63, 42.50, 67.50, 196.50, 452.93 777.50 ~
TIPS	Place the laser on the sacrum.

SPRAINS

CUSTOM	20, 5000, 10000 ~
TIPS	Soak cabbage outer leaves in hot water, wrap around sprain for 10-15 mins; try hot Epsom salts bath; Combine almond oil and garlic oil and massage area.

STIFF MUSCLES

CUSTOM	(general) 320, 328, 304, 300, 240, 160, 776, 728, 1800, 125, 80, 40, 20, 6000 ~ (neck) 4.9, 6, 9.19 ~ (shoulder) 10000, 727, 766, 20 ~
TIPS	Apply compress of apple cider vinegar to help draw out excess lactic acid.

TENNIS ELBOW

CUSTOM	0.08, 7.25, 50, 62.50, 93.50, 322.53, 475.03, 527, 667, 987.23 ~
TIPS	R.I.C.E = Rest injury immediately; Ice area as soon as possible; Compress the area; Elevate elbow above the heart; Alternate heat and cold pack

PAIN:

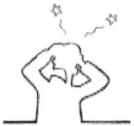

ABDOMINAL PAIN

CUSTOM	10000, 3, 3000, 95 ~
TIPS	In the pelvic area, find the middle of the crease where the leg joins the trunk of the body. Press firmly with fingers and hold for 3-5 minutes.

ACUTE PAIN

CUSTOM	3000, 95, 10000, 1550, 802, 880, 787, 727, 690, 666 ~
TIPS	Find the joint where thumb and index finger meet. Apply pressure until you find the most tender spot. Massage or hold firmly for 3-5 minutes.

BUNION PAIN

CUSTOM	20 ~
TIPS	Massage regularly with olive oil laced with little turmeric.

HEADACHES

CUSTOM	304, 144, 1.2, 520, 5.8, 6.3, 7.83, 3000, 650, 625, 600 ~ 0.16, 0.55, 0.95, 7.50, 22.50, 42.50, 96.50, 275.52, 515.70, 650 ~ (Biliary headache) 8.5, 3.5 ~
TIPS	Using thumbs or fingers, press firmly and slowly beneath base of skull in the hollow on both sides. Tilt head back, close eyes and take slow, deep breaths. Hold for 2-3 minutes.

MIGRAINE

CUSTOM	10 ~
TIPS	Place the laser on Sphenoid (temples above ears); Crush some cloves of garlic. Put two drops of the juice in the nostril relevant to the pain; Paste of garlic can be applied on the affected side of the forehead for 5 to 6 minutes.

NEURALGIA

CUSTOM	(General) - 95, 833, 10000 ~
	Intercostal (between ribs) - 802 ~
	Trigeminal (facial) - 880 ~
TIPS	Add a pinch of cayenne pepper to olive oil and massage (test first for sensitivity).

PAIN OF INFECTION

CUSTOM	95, 3000, 880, 1550, 802, 787, 776, 7279 ~
TIPS	If the pain is localised, try using the probe (Red for surface issues; Infra-red for more dense tissue).

PAIN RELIEF

CUSTOM	304, 6000, 3000, 666, 80 ~
	666, 3000, 95, 666, 80 ~
TIPS	If the pain is localised, try using the probe (Red for surface issues; Infra-red for more dense tissue).

PAINFUL MENSTRUATION
(DYSMENORRHEA)

CUSTOM	26, 4.9, 1550, 880, 802, 787, 727, 465 ~
	(Cramps) 26 ~
	10000, 880, 787, 727, 26 ~
	(Cramping and Nausea) 72, 95, 190, 880, 832, 787, 727, 20, 4.9 ~
TIPS	Take 1-2 tbsp flax seed during menstrual cycle.

SKIN ISSUES:

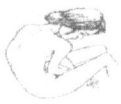

ACNE

CUSTOM	2720, 2170, 1800, 1600, 1550, 1552, 1500, 802, 880, 787, 727, 564, 778 ~
TIPS	Drink wheatgrass juice daily; Massage Milk of Magnesia on affected area, rinse off; Apply aloe vera gel; Apply paste of plain yoghurt and fine oatmeal. Leave to dry before rinsing off.

BLISTER

CUST OM	465, 660, 690, 727, 787, 880, 10000
TIPS	Resist the temptation to pop the blister; Smear some calendula ointment or pure aloe vera gel and keep clean, lightly covered with gauze; Relieve itchiness by covering with cold damp flannel.

BRUISES

CUSTOM	2720, 10000, 110, 9.1 ~
TIPS	Apply a rag soaked in comfrey tea; Try Witch Hazel; Take Arnica.

BURNS

CUSTOM	10000, 880, 787, 727, 465, 200, 190 ~
TIPS:	*NB: Not for the squeamish:* Moisten a cotton wool pad with your own fresh urine and place immediately on the burn. (Omit if you are on medication as urine will contain toxins); Try aloe vera.

CUTS

CUSTOM	20 ~
TIPS	Turmeric is a natural antiseptic and antibiotic. Apply directly on cut to stop bleeding and pain.

113

ECZEMA

CUSTOM	10000, 5000, 2720, 2008, 2180, 2128, 1550, 802, 707, 787, 727, 664, 120, 20, 9.19 ~ 916, 770, 415 ~ 1550, 802, 787, 730.2, 690 ~ (Dermatitis) - 0.03, 0.41, 0.62, 0.95, 7.50, 125.31, 387.50, 682.10, 822.06, 925.93 ~
TIPS	Sunbathing is beneficial; Coconut oil is a good moisturiser; Apply paste of nutmeg and water; Mix some tea tree oil in Vaseline and apply.

WOUNDS

CUSTOM	2720, 880, 787, 727, 220, 190, 40, 20 ~ (General antiseptic) 10000, 855, 787, 760, 777, 660, 450 ~
TIPS	See above (Cuts); See below (Infections – General/ Medicine Cabinet).

STOMACH ISSUES:

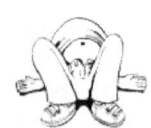

CONSTIPATION

CUSTOM	1550, 880, 802, 832, 787, 776, 422, 727, 20 ~
TIPS	Ensure your intake of water is at least 6-8 glasses; Try 2-4 tsps castor oil; First thing in the morning, on an empty stomach, drink some water that has been kept in a copper container.

DIAORRHOEA

CUSTOM	727, 787, 800, 880 ~
TIPS	Try PARASITES frequencies below: Drink carrot soup; Take a glass of water with 1 tsp apple cider vinegar each meal.

FLATULENCE

CUSTOM	1550, 880, 802, 787, 727, 465 ~
TIPS	Chew peppermint after meals; Soak fresh ginger slices in lime juice and chew after meals.

HYPERACIDITY - STOMACH

CUSTOM	20, 230 ~
TIPS	Eat bananas, watermelon, cucumbers; Suck on cloves.

INDIGESTION (DYSPEPSIA)

CUSTOM	10000, 880, 1550, 832, 800, 787, 727, 465, 444, 20, 125, 95, 72, 4.9 ~
TIPS	Take 2 tsps white vinegar with meals; Eat papaya or fresh pineapple after meals.

MOTION SICKNESS

CUSTOM	625, 600, 465, 648, 1865, 522 ~ 0.15, 0.23, 0.68, 0.83, 72.52, 137.57, 292.61, 537.30, 822.59, 921.05 ~
TIPS	Sit in the front; Focus on the distance, keeping your eyes on the horizon.

NAUSEA AND CRAMPING

CUSTOM	95, 832, 727, 20, 95, 72, 20, 3.9, 450, 802, 1552, 832, 422 ~
TIPS	Take few drops of clove oil; Drink peppermint or chamomile tea; Apply pressure between thumb and forefinger.

PARASITES

CUSTOM	20, 47, 60, 64, 72, 96, 112, 120, 125, 128, 152, 240, 334, 422, 442, 465, 524, 642, 644, 651, 669, 666, 676, 688, 690, 712, 728, 732, 740, 751, 770,780, 784, 787, 800, 802, 854, 880, 1360, 1550, 1552, 1840, 1862, 1864, 1998, 2008, 2112, 2128, 3176, 4412, 10000 ~
TIPS	Run the programme daily, several times a day, to kill the parasites in all its life cycles. Take castor oil - follow the directions on the bottle; Eat raw garlic; Drink pomegranate juice daily; Drink coconut water daily.

MEDICINE CABINET ESSENTIALS:

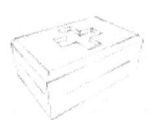

COLD SORES

CUSTOM	464, 1488 (for 15 minutes): then 1489, 1500, 1550, 1577, 1900 ~
TIPS	Hold cut garlic on the sore; Press small amount of salt on the sore (painful but effective); Hold ice cube on sore for as long as possible.

FATIGUE - GENERAL

CUSTOM	428, 424, 664, 660, 464, 125, 120, 95, 72, 20, 444, 1865, 10000, 5000 ~
TIPS	Identify what long or short-term stress might be the cause.

FEVER

CUSTOM	(Various causes) - 880, 800, 832, 422, 2112, 787, 727, 20 ~
TIPS	Remember: Fevers help the body fight infection and eliminate toxins; Drink lots of water; Take cool baths; Wear cotton socks soaked in white vinegar.

FOOD POISONING

CUSTOM	727, 787, 880, 10000 ~
TIPS	To kill bacteria - Sweeten the juice of 4 lemons and drink straight; Try half a cup of Colloidal Silver; To eliminate gas - Try activated charcoal; To line the stomach – Eat sweetened stewed apples; Try natural, unflavoured yoghurt.

FOOT BLISTERS

CUSTOM	10000, 880, 787, 727, 465 ~
TIPS	Soften by soaking for 15 minutes in warm water; Apply aloe vera; Smear castor oil or Vaseline and leave overnight; Apply a paste of apple cider vinegar and mashed raw onions.

HANGOVER

CUSTOM	10000, 522, 146 ~
TIPS	Drink lots of water; Eat citrus fruits (Vitamin C) in the morning; Eat raw cabbage; Take hot bath to drain away toxins.

HAYFEVER

CUSTOM	(Some types) 880, 787, 727, 20 ~
TIPS	Include regular intake of honey in diet to desensitise to pollen; Smear Vaseline around nostrils to catch pollen before it is breathed in.

HAEMORRHOIDS

CUSTOM	20, 727, 800, 880 ~
TIPS	Increase fibre and water intake; Alternate hot and cold compress to the area; Use pad or absorbent probe soaked with Witch Hazel.

INFECTIONS - GENERAL

CUSTOM	880, 802, 786, 728, 95, 72, 48, 20, 5500, 676, 422 ~
TIPS	Apply crushed <u>onions</u> on wound, leave up to one hour to draw out infection, rinse, repeat as necessary. Apply a dab of <u>honey</u>, cover with gauze. It will emit hydrogen peroxide and antibiotic properties; Sprinkle <u>Turmeric</u> directly on wound, cover with bandage. It will clean out bacteria, stop bleeding and help control infections; Sprinkle some <u>ginger</u> on wound, cover with bandage, change as necessary. Ginger is antiseptic and cleans wounds.

INSOMNIA

CUSTOM	3, 7.83, 10, 1550, 1500, 880, 802, 6000, 304 ~
TIPS	Place the laser on the Sphenoid (temples above ears); Keep a bedside notepad to write down any thoughts keeping you awake; Learn to meditate.

VERUCCA

CUSTOM	644, 767, 797, 877, 953, 173, 787 ~
TIPS	Place square of banana skin on the verucca; or cotton wool ball dipped in vinegar, or juice of a crushed onion, and leave overnight; Try Tea Tree oil.

BODY SYSTEMS / STATES (STIMULATE / STRENGTHEN):

BODY SYSTEM	FREQUENCY
Adrenal Function	1335 Hz
Endocrine System Function	1537 Hz
Immune System	835 Hz
Nervous System	764 Hz
Lymph System	676 Hz
Increased **Lymph** System Circulation	15 Hz
Pineal Function	480 Hz
Pituitary Function	635 Hz
Thyroid **Function**	763 Hz

BODY SYSTEM	FREQUENCY
Colon Function	635 Hz
Liver Function	751 Hz
Kidney Function	625 Hz
Heart Function	696 Hz
Pancreas Function	654 Hz

BODY SYSTEM	FREQUENCY
Healing of **Nerves**	2.0 Hz
Healing of **Bones**	7.0 Hz
Healing of **Ligaments**	9.7 Hz
Healing of **Muscles**	13.5 Hz
Healing of **Capillaries**	15.2 Hz
Reduce excess fluid - **Joints** & **Tissues**	24.3 Hz

BODY SYSTEM	FREQUENCY
Blood Circulation	337 Hz
Increased **Blood Flow / Circulation**	17 Hz
Blood Pressure	15 Hz
Red Blood Cell Production	1524 Hz
White Blood Cell Production	1434 Hz
Calcium Metabolism	328 Hz
DNA Integrity	528 Hz
RNA Integrity	637 Hz

BODY STATES	FREQUENCY
Clarity of Thought / Mental Function	35 Hz
Stabilization of **Emotional States**	15 Hz
Clearing Emotional **Trauma / Energy Blocks**	15 Hz
Balancing of **Spiritual Well-Being**	1565 Hz
Reduction **Chemical Sensitivity**	440 Hz
Reduction **Electrical Sensitivity**	657 Hz
Induce **Sleep**	80 Hz

Experimental Frequencies
Source: www.Stenulson.net

CHAKRA SYSTEM	FREQUENCY
Root	3.8 - 4.3 Hz
Sacral	5.6 - 6.2 Hz
Solar Plexus	9.8 - 10.2 Hz
Heart	11.8 - 12.2 Hz
Throat	15.8 -16.2 Hz
Third Eye	90.0 - 98.0 Hz
Crown	960.0 Hz

Source: Kelly Research Technologies

NB: The author cannot ascertain that any of the sources or frequencies listed are either valid or accurate. The reader accepts full responsibility for any frequency programming.

HEALING CRISIS

Cold lasers have a detoxifying effect on the cells and tissue. Sometimes due to the quantity of bacteria released, and our system discharging toxins faster than the body can release them, the body goes into what is known as a healing crisis. The signs and symptoms of this crisis, or '*Herxheimer Reaction*,' can be identical to the illness itself (eg. fatigue, headaches; muscular stiffness, general aches and pains, sore throat, indigestion, increased blood pressure, increased heart beat, etc.) and may come after you've been feeling good and energised. As a consequence, you may doubt the effectiveness of your laser, or feel that it is causing you more harm than good. Actually, these are signs that the body's defence system and elimination channels – kidneys, lungs, digestion, liver, lymph, sweat glands - are working to kill off and disgorge microbes. The clearing of toxins and impurities is all part of the healing process.

Commonly, a frequency is administered for 3 minutes – but this could be either too long or insufficient, depending on how the detox is affecting you. Start with shorter sessions (30 seconds is OK) and gradually build up. After this initial period, you are your own guide. In terms of how often to have sessions, this also depends on your rate of detox. Three times per day or once every three days might be your limit. Though after a session you may feel sluggish or tired; over the next few days you will gradually feel renewed and ready for another session. The above advice, however, is just a precaution, and may not apply to you. Not everyone feels worse before they feel better.

NB: Continue your sessions even after all your symptoms have gone. Germs are pleomorphic – ie they have a life cycle with different developmental stages, and you are aiming to eliminate them at every stage.

WHAT TO DO:

- Drink plenty of filtered water, increase your normal amount – tea, coffee and fizzy or carbonated drinks do not count as water!
- Eat fresh fruit, vegetables and whole grains
- Take Vitamin C, a great detoxifier
- Exercise daily, according to your ability
- Stimulate your lymph system by dry-brushing your body and/or rebounding
- Take time out, rest when necessary, reduce your workload
- Bask in sunshine, walk in nature, engage in activities that you love.
- If necessary, reduce the intensity of your treatment

NB: Use common sense. If at any time you are concerned, seek medical advice.

HELPFUL RIFE REFERENCES

To help you on your journey of discovery, I have included a number of sites below. Do your own research to obtain specific frequencies to meet your own health and wellness challenges. You will find that you are opening the door on a wonderful world of optimism and self-empowerment.

NB: The authors below do not claim that any of the frequencies they list will diagnose, treat, cure or otherwise affect the outcome of any disease or condition. *Always* take responsibility for your own health.

NAME	INFORMATION	SITE / LINK
Nenah Sylver, PhD	*The Rife Handbook* + frequency information	www.nenahsylver.com http://www.nenahsylver.com/description-and-contents.html
Richard Lloyd, PhD	Extensive list of frequencies	www.royalrife.com http://royalrife.com/freq_list.pdf
Dr Hulda Clark	Information on parasites + frequency list	www.huldaclarkzappers.com http://www.huldaclarkzappers.com/frequency.pdf
Stone Circle	Master List of Rife Frequencies	www.stonecirclealternatives.com http://www.stonecirclealternatives.com/rifeail.pdf
Stone Circle	Reverse list of frequencies – useful for cross-referencing	www.stonecirclealternatives.com http://www.stonecirclealternatives.com/rifefreq.pdf
Electro-Herbalism	Frequencies + reference to *The Electroherbalism Frequency Lists Book*	www.electroherbalism.com http://www.electroherbalism.com/Bioelectronics/FrequenciesandAnecdotes/CAFL.htm
Altered-States	Comprehensive list of frequencies	www.altered-states.net http://altered-states.net/barry/newsletter135/frequecies.htm

With the exception of Nenah Sylver, most of the ABC frequencies I have used in this Handbook have been sourced from the above websites.

You can also find these links on my website: **www.iheartmylaser.com**

AND FINALLY...

How Chronic Back Pain Led to My Laser Love Affair!

I had never considered myself a 'back pain sufferer.' Like most people, on and off I'd experienced the occasional ache in the lumbago region. I also recall an episode several years ago when I developed a really painful stress-related knot in my lower back and had to have it massaged out by a professional masseuse. But I wasn't familiar with the kind of long-term incapacitating condition that has some people crawling around on all fours, weeping for morphine. In my work as a healer, I often see clients with back-related issues who can barely make it up the steps, never mind haul themselves onto the massage couch. And that's with the help of strong painkillers. One day I received a phone call from a lady* who was sobbing so uncontrollably I could hardly hear what she was saying. Eventually, I made out, *'I know it's a Sun(sob)day, but I'm in such (sob) pain. Please (sob), please (sob), can you see me (sob) now!'* Little did I realise a year later, that I might be on the phone to several alternative practitioners on the verge of similar tears.

125

One fine day I was out on one of my usual shopping sprees. Ladies, you know the kind. You pop into the supermarket for two specific little items, and step out with ten bags weighing several kilos in weight. I remember feeling the pressure of those bags in my hip joints and lower back muscles. But I struggled home, reprimanding myself for overdoing it, yet again unable to resist the lure of the 'Buy 2 Get 1 Free.' That night I felt a distinct twinge in the base of my spine, a warning. The next morning I woke up in pure agony. There was nothing I could do to alleviate the grating ache in my groin, the bone-deep stiffness in my lower back and the red hot spasms that came in pulsating immobilising waves. Each wave wrenched an involuntary cry from me. I'd grip the nearest thing to hand, and freeze. From that paralysed position, the fear of being jolted a micro millimetre was greater than the fear of Death. As if it could get any worse, the pain progressively became more unbearable.

Eventually, I could neither stand, sit, kneel, crouch, step nor lie down without triggering another bout of throbbing seizures. Self-healing was out of the question. It was impossible for me to focus on anything other than the searing pain. I couldn't believe how my life had changed so quickly, so drastically - one minute a reckless load-bearing shopper, the next a crippled invalid. When the spasms began coming every few minutes and I could hardly breathe (like childbirth, but without benefits), my partner took the matter in hand and decided to drive me to Accident and Emergency. However, it took longer for me to negotiate the impossibility of getting in and out of the car than it took to make the 20 minute trip to the hospital for the two-hour wait. By then, I was so rigid with pain I couldn't/wouldn't allow the doctor to examine me. It was a Sunday afternoon, probably past this medic's lunchtime. Though kindly, he had seen it all before. He very quickly gave up on the examination (and me) and packed me off with a large plastic bag rattling with enough pills to paralyse a horse.

Being a pure soul (no alcohol, no cigarettes, no drugs, no caffeine), I wanted nothing to do with those chemicals. Yet, it took extreme willpower not to cram my mouth and swallow the lot. Sanity prevailed, and I restricted my dosage to the minimum. A very wise decision, as it turned out. The chemicals barely took the edge off the pain, but were pretty effective in stripping the lining of my virgin gut. I now had excruciating abdominal pain to match the excruciating back pain. My poor children became my unpaid carers. Before going off to school, they'd coax mum in and out of the shower while she took fearful, ginger steps. I would wince in anticipation of every movement as they assisted in putting on my clothes. My partner washed, cooked, cleaned and house-husbanded for several weeks as I was capable of little more than shuffling around ghost-like, wearing a housecoat and a pitiful grimace. During this period I admit that one of my vain preoccupations was to count the appearance of each new frown line. My low point was one afternoon when I was alone in the house and unable to lower myself into a comfortable sitting or lying position without setting off pain alarm bells. I pigeon-paced back and forth from the kitchen to the back room for an unending 2 HOURS till the family returned home.

During the first two weeks I spent over £600 seeing or being seen by the following: Reiki Grand Master; Gigong Master; Distance Healer; Energy Healer; Acupuncturist 1; Acupuncturist 2; Chiropractor 1 (whose x-ray diagnosed my condition, ankylosing spondilitis); Chiropractor 2; EFT/Reiki practitioner. Then there was my family and army of practitioner friends: Fros, who offered a session of Bowen therapy; Rachel, who arrived with her Scenar bio-feedback device; Caroline, who intuitively scanned my body and came up with important insights; Robert, a client, friend and EFT newbie, who tapped surrogately for me; my daughter who ferried me to and from various therapists and healers. I even had wonderful seven year old Clara visit specially to put her hand on my back and order the pain to 'Be GONE!' Each one of these amazing people helped, soothed and cared for me, and sometimes (due, I think, to their loving attention) the pain would reduce. But the main hellishness stubbornly gripped my back like a rusty vice. It was confounding, why no-one was able to help me definitively, when I had helped so many of my clients suffering from similar agonies.

One day I called up a guy with a reputation for being a healer (one of the few with website testimonials) who had written a book, *'It's OK Not To Be OK.'* I wasn't sure it was OK, but I had begrudgingly come to the conclusion that the root issue causing the pain, was in my subconscious. There was something deeply emotional that I was refusing to address in my life. The pain represented my 'stuckness.' I kind of figured what the issue was, but I needed someone experienced enough to see through my willful denial and steer me forward. As an EFT (Emotional Freedom Technique) practitioner, I'm familiar with the mental tricks that clients bring to my door. *'Of course I want to lose weight – I am so ready!'* (But what if I achieve a size 12 only to put the weight on again? What if I lose my attractive bubbly personality? What if being slim makes me visible*?); 'Of course I want to go for that dream job I've waited all my life for, are you crazy?'* (But what if they hate me and turn me down? What if I'm not up to it? Why risk the rejection, the failure, the shame?); *'Of course I love myself!'* (I just hate my hips/acne/bum/voice/bra size). Over the years, I have honed the ability to cut through my clients' protestations, guiding them to the heart of the unconscious self-sabotage causing their emotional/physical manifestations. However, this also means that I am extra-adept at pulling the wool over the eyes of anyone whose task it is to uncover my own little nest of vipers.

My therapeutic saviour, Arram Kong, turned up. Little did I know that he would also double as my guardian angel. He waited for several minutes as I negotiated and re-negotiated how to mount my own massage table without triggering those frayed nerve endings. I finally managed it and was surprised to be asked to lie on my front. Strange, for an EFT session, I thought. But I wasn't the one in charge, so who was I to argue? My suspicions started to grow, however, when rather than take my hand to tap my acupressure points, I heard him briskly unzipping a bag. He instructed me to 'just lie there' as he was about to try out a 'new light machine' on me. To say I was annoyed is putting it ever so mildly. I'd psyched myself up to confront my demons but instead of getting on with demon-slaying, this man was placing some flashing gimmick-thingy on my back. Well, the surprise was on me. Several minutes in, I released an unexpected spontaneous sigh. In no time I noticed my breathing becoming deeper, more regular. I could feel my entire body gently lengthening… unwinding… relaxing. I even started to drift off a little, forgetting my guarded vigil for the pain. Arram asked me to carefully try to arch my back. Without even questioning the wisdom of this, I did, and found that I could! I'm not sure how long the process took, but the end result was that I was able to ease myself off the massage couch with barely any assistance and walk around the room, pain-free for the first time in two weeks. I even dared, and was able, to TOUCH MY TOES! The pain-mask I'd been wearing cracked as I broke into a smile of utter disbelief.

My family and some visiting friends looked up in astonishment when I glided, without the usual halting, rusty movements, into the dining room. Everyone commented how alive my face looked, as though something awful had lifted from it. That evening I had a seated meal for the first time in weeks. I joined in conversation, laughed, and felt human again, sitting in company for nearly two hours without so much as a reminder twitch. I was joyous, grateful and fearless as I went to bed that night.

The next morning - Wham! - the pain returned, hitting me in the lower back like a runaway heavy-goods train. It was every bit as excruciating as all the times before. But rather than losing all hope, I intuitively knew that something imperceptible had shifted somewhere inside of me. I also knew that I had to have that laser on my back again. Arram invited me to a laser meeting that happened to be in London that week. I arrived at the venue slumped like a broken doll in the back of my friend's car. During the entire meeting, whilst the person at the front and delivered his presentation, I was on Arram's laser. Its effects weren't as dramatic as the first time, but I was confident that it was working at a deeper, more profound level. So much so, that I made the decision to buy my own laser. I had a real gut instinct that this purchase would never see the bottom of my wicker-basket.

It took a while, but each day I felt I was making progress. First the abdominal pain went, then the central lower back pain, and slowly the pain either side of my spine dissolved. My life began to return to normal. After all I'd been through, one day, I even caught myself being that reckless shopper again! If ever I needed a sign of healing, that was it. After three months, what remained was a vague reminder of pain in my lower back. Five months later, I was like new again. As I write this, a year on, my back is still good. This is in contrast to people I know suffering from the same condition who are on daily painkillers, constantly fluctuating between bad days and excruciating days – FOR YEARS! I try to tell them and everyone I meet about this wonderful device and my love affair with it. However, not everyone is willing or able to believe that a moulded plastic gizmo can contain magic and transform an actual medical condition.

My laser has now become my silent assistant when I'm working with clients, and I'm in no doubt that it enhances my usual results. It also saves my energies. After long hours seeing clients, sometimes I'm too exhausted or indifferent to administer to my own family. These days, I simply tell them to get on the laser. As for myself, I use it daily for minor ailments, for health maintenance and, of course, for anti-ageing! I LOVE my laser SO much, I remember (rather like a first-time mum) panicking the moment I first held it – what if I lost it, how on earth would I cope? Then I relaxed and reassured myself, 'I'd buy another one. No questions asked.'

The body is always communicating with us. There is always a message in the imbalance, the disease, the disorder. So, what did I discover about myself in relation to my own suffering? Nothing I didn't already know at a deeper level. Pain and disease in the body is usually a metaphor for what is happening in one's life, changes that need to be made, I tell my clients all the time. The lower back has its own message. It points to unconscious beliefs related to Support, or lack of it. Or, perceived lack of it.

In my life, my record reads that I have a tendency to feel that I have to 'do it all,' that I am the only one who can 'do it right,' that I can't trust anyone around me to deliver in the way that only I can. And that should I trust or believe in another person to the extent that I believe in myself, I will only be let down. Who could blame my outlook when disappointment has been my experience countless times in my life? So, given that I won't allow anyone the chance to disprove that I am right about my beliefs, it's no surprise that the major emotion that arises in me is a feeling of being unsupported. However, during my illness I was forced to examine this perception of myself, acknowledging that its seeds originate from a particular childhood crisis. My reality at this time had been that I couldn't rely on the One Source of true support - the Universe. How could I, when it had shown exactly the opposite of support, by taking my mother away from me? This was my unconscious belief.

My mother died a few days before my 13th birthday. It was a shock that was too enormous to absorb, and the impact didn't properly hit me until decades later. At that tender age, showing little emotions, I took it upon myself to head up the family. I became very proficient at depending on Me, 'making it happen'; becoming a 'do-er'; a 'giver,' never a 'receiver.' I had my head down and didn't see that there was a lesson I had to learn that kept showing up, time and time again. The lesson I failed to acknowledge, despite the numerous opportunities presented to me, was this: in life there are many occasions to receive, to accept support, and one must be gracious and open to them. If you are blind to that support, you also become blind to the joys of life. Resentment, blame and judgement start creeping into your way of seeing things. Eventually, these negative emotions settle as subtle cellular contractions in the body, depriving that particular area of life-giving energy. Over the years, as more disappointments are experienced, attracted by a restricted way of viewing the world, these negative emotions gradually weaken that targeted (vulnerable) part of your body – in my case, my lower back.

When I became incapacitated, forced to depend on everyone around me - for everything - the scales, very slowly, began to fall from my eyes. There was no choice but to allow the support I was being given – from being dressed, to being driven, to being shopped for, to being cooked for, to accepting sympathetic company, to even being helped across the road! The latter occurred when it became necessary for me to see my doctor. This was due to the hospital-medication-inflicted gut-ache I was suffering. I made the short journey unaccompanied as the family were at work and school. The thought of crossing three roads to the surgery filled me with terror. Every step was fraught with the very real possibility of my back jarring and going into spasm. What if an impatient driver accelerated when I was only halfway across the road? What if the pain became so bad I could neither stop nor continue walking? What if...? By the time I got to the third road I had become a nervous wreck. I called out to a young girl. She held my hand and pigeon-stepped with me to the other side. Accepting help had become a strange and uncomfortable 'first' experience for me. It felt like using a muscle that I'd forgotten I was born with. That muscle was stiff, de-oxygenated, self-conscious, and painful to move. Behind it there was the usual belief that no-one could 'do' any of 'it' exactly like me. Even the girl who helped me cross the road, didn't fully appreciate my condition, walking that millisecond too fast for my either ability or my liking. My inner protestations made perfect sense, I had been accustomed to telling myself. After all, there *is* only one of me in the entire Universe! But, then... that goes for you, too. *Everyone*, not just me, has a uniqueness, a value, to offer to this world. And appreciation, gratitude and acknowledgement of each special relationship, each new experience, is what opens the magical door on our very real participation in life. Slowly, I began to see the gift in my illness, and to see that a long time ago, upon the death of my mother, I had unconsciously closed that door.

During my bad back phase, I discovered Iwin, a wise and wonderfully talented Chinese acupuncturist who was among those that came to my aid. She explained that I'd accumulated an excess of cold energy (chi) as a result of not protecting myself from the negative energies of my clients. As someone for whom healing came intuitively and relatively late in life, I had never learned the rituals of protection. Neither did I believe in them. Iwin, however, a healer herself, advised that these rituals were essential if I wasn't to deplete my own energies and expose myself to problems. I began to see that she might be right – in a way. Though I still don't subscribe to the idea of 'fear-based' protection, she opened my eyes to how I was viewing the world: in order to maintain the amazing results I'd been getting, along with the many glowing client testimonials, I had indeed been using reserves of my own energy. With hindsight, it became clear that this was the same trust issue, feeding into my belief of being short-changed by the Universe. I was trying too hard, believing that unless I gave *everything* to each and every client (Once, because I was determined to achieve the *right* results for my client, the session lasted a whole 3 hours!), I would 'fail' each time. I distrusted the abundance of Universal energy that surrounds and supports us, not fully allowing myself to become One with All That Is. In other words, I was failing to step into the effortlessness, the boundlessness, the magnificence, of my true power. No wonder the therapists I contacted were unable to help me. Not even the Qigong Master's solid reputation had an iota of impact on my agony. I remember seeing a flash of distress in his otherwise qi-focused eyes and asking in-beween howls of agony, 'Am I your worst nightmare?' Neither of us realised that it wasn't a one-session wonder that would save me, it was *time*. And reflection. And that's when laser technology entered my life. Its timing could not have been more perfect.

Each day I used my laser, I sank into *zero-point*, a delicious sea of calm and tranquillity that allowed me to float above all the minor everyday undercurrents of disappointment, annoyance and irritation, and to go with the *flow* of life. It was this *flow* (combined with the specific frequencies resonating with my condition) that became my healing force. From this place I was able to begin my self-healing. Forgiveness and acceptance of the past played an important part, including mentally releasing that 13 year old from her vow of isolation and fierce independence. Today, I am so much stronger, and feel that I now have the back that I deserve.

That doesn't mean that I've 'arrived' at some place of finite welcome. And neither have I lost my powerful ambition. I'm still learning, still growing, still going at my own pace, towards the Light of my own awakening. That's my prerogative, that's my purpose on this earth. As it is yours. The difference, though, is that I am now *listening*. All the time. When my back communicates with me and tells me that I am out of balance, I have to ask, *where, how, when,* with *what* or *whom*? At this point it's usually an indication for me to reach for my laser and, with its assistance, meditatively welcome the answers. I realise now, that my reckless shopping moment wasn't the <u>cause</u> of what happened to me. It was the mere tipping point; the straw that broke what had become the most vulnerable part of me – my back. But, just as importantly, it directed me to where I am now –

connecting with you, dear Reader. It has also led me to conclude that there were more profound reasons for my journey of suffering. Those reasons were three-fold:

1. to learn an important lesson about life, relationships, joy – and letting go
2. to discover, through Arram Kong, the miracle of my amazing cold laser
3. to lovemylaserSOmuch! this Handbook would effortlessly write itself and provide Light and understanding to all those who read it.

Namaste.

*Incidentally, the lady left my house completely free of pain. She later phoned to tell me that her astonished GP, who had been treating her for months and had previously signed her off work, wanted my telephone number! Not only had she come off the pain-killers immediately, soon afterwards she had been able to return to her job as a bus driver. And not long after that, I was told that she walked, not hobbled, down the aisle.

Sketch/Cartoon images (Rights):

Supandi Wijaya
Robodread
Bea Kraus
Pzaxe
Colin Cramm
Francois Barret
John Takai
Ioan Panaite
123RF.COM